PROCESSING   REVIT

STRONG   I HAVE MORE ROOM!

MEDITATING   PEACEFUL

MORE ENLIGHTENED

CONTEMPLATIVE   RELIEVED

CONTINUALLY AMAZED

EUPHORIC   EFFERVESCENT

ANTICIPATION & JOY   STRONG

CLARITY   CONNECTED TO LIFE

CONFIDENT   EXPANDED

BLISSED OUT   BIGGER   CALM

NATURAL HIGH   AERATED

HUNGRY   INSIGHTFUL

DRAINED & FILLED   RELAXED

The Silent, Deep Universe
in My Teen Brain

Hey there, Denis!

My husband David and I attended your breathwork seminar at the yoga studio in Medford yesterday. It was a chance to rub shoulders and talk to people so much more like us than the previous collection of folks we have shared our incarnation with so far. You, the facilitator from Montana, are the fellow that Steve and Mary Caroll* met when they were on their annual trek to the West, something many of us from the East do to connect with the pioneer spirit.

Originally from the East Coast, you saw Montana in 1989 and never looked back. You father was a doctor and the first year or two of your college education was in pre-med, so massage and breathwork seemed like natural choices for someone who started out as a hippie.

After a few hours of lectures on the physiology of breathing and some evaluations to determine our own breathing efficiency (or lack of it), we settled down for the work at hand. Led by a CD with the breathing done by a coach, we all proceeded to follow the breathing rhythm for twenty minutes or so.

We were on our backs, eyes closed, blankets upon us. I thought I'd fall asleep, but it's called breath-*work* for a reason—it was work! The breathing was fast, just under what would have led to hyperventilation. As I lay on my back with my eyes closed, it reminded me of the *corpse pose* that ends my yoga sessions.

Thinking about corpses made me think about dying, which made me think about childbirth, which made me feel like I was being birthed, which made me realize I have been born, I AM born, and will be born again, and that I am every bit as eternally alive now as I will be when I reach the Great Beyond. I felt the same could be said of everyone there in the room with me, which made me love them all so fiercely! I realized that THIS—right here and right now—is the eternal moment. This is the heaven we are all taught to wait for, which we are told is far away and will be ours only if we jump through very specific hoops. I was no longer afraid of crying in front of everyone in the room. I no longer even felt separated from them... All in the first twenty minutes!

Almost as soon as my epiphany peaked, the breathing on the CD gave way to music that sounded like a heavenly celebration, the Universe joining my teen brain in a chorus that invited me: Would I step outside of myself and join the Eternal One? Hell, yes!

The next forty minutes was an opportunity to recover from the experience—a time spent equally between laughing and crying. The phenomenal simplicity of it all split my atoms apart into a light show, a sound show. It was a chance to float and dance, to swing, bob and weave, to sail on an ocean of understanding that does not depend on my outer surroundings for existence. It has been waiting to manifest—waiting for me to cross the divide that is no larger than the atoms in which I exist. They have collected and congealed into a mass everyone calls Karen, but there is much more—and much less—to all of this.

I understood all this in one of those deep understandings that will not disappear with time, but still grow stronger and deeper, all the while quiet, silent, and deep.

— Karen Berkey • Medford, NJ

*Special thanks to my dearest friends, Stephen and Mary Carroll, from Audubon, NJ, who sponsored a major weekend of breathwork in Medford, NJ in 2007. We did TWO half-day seminars, where over 80 participants were accommodated. On one of the Carroll's Montana visits, Steve and I climbed Emigrant Peak together (11,000 feet). Lovely Mary has since passed away. Steve carries on his psychotherapy practice where he specializes in Somatic Experiencing, the work of Dr. Peter Levine as described in the article, "Getting the War Out."

Your Inner Healer simply waits
in loving innocence
for the untainted truth
carried on your Breath.

— *Steve Moesong*

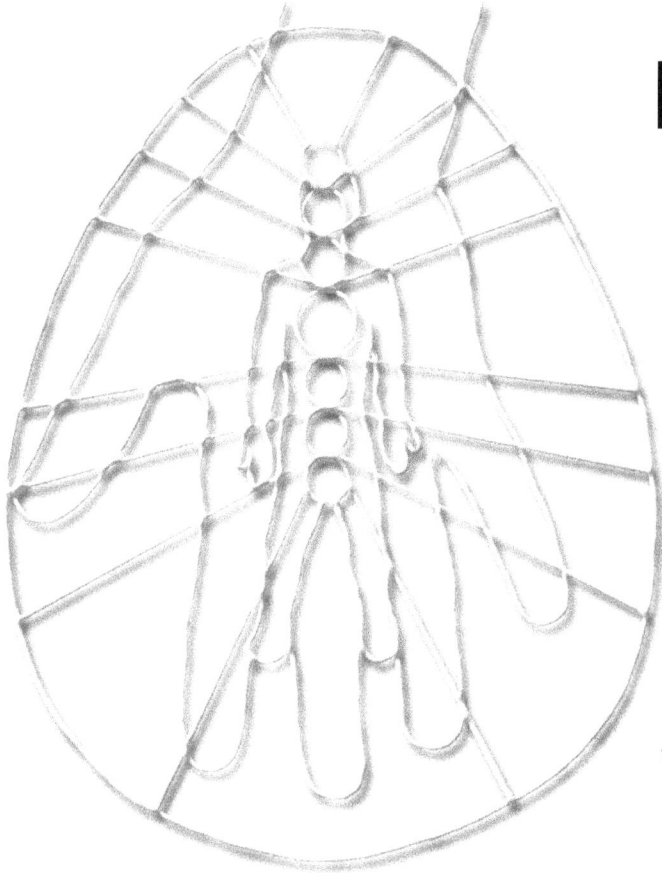

HEAL YOURSELF
with
Breath,
Light,
Sound &
Water

Denis Ouellette

with Michael Grant White • Sol Luckman • John C. Ledbetter
Debra Klein • Kevin Ryerson • Michael Richard

NATURAL LIFE
NEWS
Livingston, Montana

HEAL YOURSELF with Breath, Light, Sound and Water
Denis Ouellette

Third Edition, Copyright © 2019 by Denis Ouellette
Second Edition, Copyright © 2006 by Denis Ouellette

Part Two originally published under the title:
Rebirthing According to Spirit: Healing with Breath, Light, Sound and Water
Copyright © 1982, 1984 by Denis Ouellette

The author of this book does not, either directly or indirectly, dispense medical advice nor prescribe the use of any practice as a form of treatment for physical, mental or emotional problems without the advice of a physician or qualified health professional. The intent of the author is to offer information of a general nature to assist readers in their quest for good health and wellness. In the event that you use any of the information in this book for yourself, which is your constitutional right, the author and publisher assume no responsibility for your actions.

NOTE TO BREATHWORK FACILITATORS: Feel free to copy and use any sections of this book for your healing sessions, workshops and trainings, especially the handouts in PART THREE. Just give credit where due.

NOTE TO ALL THERAPISTS: Feel free to incorporate any materials and practices into your own modalities.

PRINT ISBN: 978-1-7339053-0-5

Cover photo: Geothermal pool at Yellowstone National Park
Photo CD: *Patterns & Textures from Yellowstone*
Copyright © 2002 by Janice McDonald

Cover design, book layout & graphics by Denis Ouellette

Revised & Updated Third Edition: March 2019 • Second Edition, June 2006
First Edition: First Printing, November 1982 • Second Printing, March 1984

Published by Natural Life News • www.NaturalLifeNews.com
739 North 11th Street • Livingston, Montana 59047
Printed in the United States of America

For additional copies write to Natural Life News
730 North 11th Street • Livingston, Montana 59047

Order online at www.IntegralBreathwork.com
or e-mail denis@wispwest.net

Your Best Friend

Early in this book Denis points out,
"Your breath can be your best friend."
Indeed I agree, because the breath has become
my closest friend and ally in life.
It is truly my constant and loving companion
as I travel the world on this journey
of awakening, healing, and growth.

Whether I want to calm down or to energize myself,
the breath is there to lend a helping hand.
If I want to focus my energies or expand my consciousness,
the breath is waiting to support me in this too.
And this is true for everyone.

Whether we want to remain closed or stuck or stagnant—
or choose to open ourselves to new feelings,
new dimensions, new realities, a new life—
the breath is more than willing to help us,
and it's already acting upon our subtle cues.

No matter what our present situation or calling in life,
no matter what our goals or dreams may be—
breathing is a force, a tool we can use,
a bridge of immense practical and spiritual benefit.

And it's just waiting for us to discover,
to explore, and to develop its power and potential.

I invite you to use this priceless gift called breath.

Dan Brulé, Los Cabos, Baja California Sur, Mexico
Author of *Just Breathe* • BreathMastery.com

CONTENTS

Introduction to the Third Edition • 2019   *iv*

Acknowledgments   *xiv*

PART ONE ~ BREATH, LIGHT, SOUND & WATER

1. *Inhale!*   *1*

2. Breathwork Stories:

    Releasing Vietnam   *5*

    Popcorn on a Stove   *6*

    Better Than Ten Therapy Sessions!   *6*

    Asthma, Arterial Fibrillation & Rebounding   *7*

3. *Are You Stuck in "Fight or Flight"?*   *8*

4. *Oxygen Is Life! It Does More Than You Think*—Michael Grant White

    Sidebar with: Daniel P. Reid   *11*

5. *Exhale!* Sidebar with: Daniel P. Reid   *14*

6. *Sound & Light: Energy Follows Thought*

    Sidebars with: Steve Guettermann & Gia Combs-Ramirez   *17*

7. *Water & Earth: Our Body* Sidebar with: Georgia Cold   *21*

8. *"Getting the War Out"*—New Paradigms for Healing Post-Traumatic Stress

    Sidebars with: Jacque Chapman, Michael Grant White, Peter A. Levine, Ph.D.,

    Louise J. Hill, Amber Ashby, Colin P. Sisson, Omraam, Diane Yankelevitz   *24*

PART TWO ~ NEW LIGHT ON ANCIENT HEALING

9. Preface to the 2006 Edition   *36*

10. Introduction to the 1982 Edition   *41*

ANCIENT HEALING TEMPLE—through Debra Klein   *43*

11. *You Will Fly to the Stars*—by Mother Mary   *44*

12. *Breathwork's Ancient History*—by Cochise   *46*

13. *Essene Breathwork Practices*—by Mother Mary   *55*

14. *Native American Medicine*—by Cochise   *57*

15. Questions & Answers—by Cochise   *58*

SELF-HEALING & LIFE EXTENSION—through Kevin Ryerson   *66*

16. *Physiology of Breathwork & Chakra Work*—by John the Divine   *67*

17. Questions & Answers—by John the Divine   *73*

18. *On Life Extension* with Questions & Answers—by Tom McPherson   *79*

THE ESSENE REBIRTH—through Michael Richard   *86*

19. *Essene Rebirth & Breathwork Guidelines*—by Katherine the Healer   *88*

20. *The Essene Rebirth*—by Katherine the Healer   *93*

21. *Teaching the Light*—by John the Baptist   *96*

Notes to Part Two   *102*

PART THREE ~ BREAKTHROUGHS!   105

22. More Breathwork Stories:

    A New Beginning for Me   106

    Young Indian Brave   107

    Who Is That? Is That You?   107

    They Were OK   109

    Adele's Communion   110

    Let Go and Forgive   112

ARTICLES

23 *An Ode to Massage*—Lessons from a Lifetime of Body Tune-Ups   114

24. *Tetany & Gentle Breathwork*—Denis Ouellette & Michael White

    Sidebars with: Leon Chatow, ND, Tom Goode, ND, & Dan Brulé   118

25. *Working with Difficult Cases: Medications, Detox Symptoms*

    & Chi Activation—Denis Ouellette, Michael White & J. Michael Wood

    Sidebars with: Daniel P. Reid & Joy Manné, Ph.D.   125

26. *Sound, Intention & Genetic Healing*—Sol Luckman   130

27. *The Earth's & Our Body's Health-Enhancing Electric Fields*

    —John C. Ledbetter   135

28. *Fatigue—Its Cause & Antidote*—D.O. Harrell, MD

    Excerpts from *Deep Breathing & Nerve Force*—Paul von Boeckmann   141

29. *The Continuum*   148

APPENDIX   151

30. OPTIMAL BREATHING®—Michael White

    Optimal Breathing Self-Test, Parts 1 & 2   152

    Supporting a More Optimal Breathing Pattern:

    The Pear + The Cone = The Wave • Squeeze & Breathe Exercise   156

31. INTEGRAL BREATHWORK™

    Seminar Flyers, Agenda, Registration Packet, Evaluation Form, etc.   158

    Our Nervous Systems   164

    What to Do • What to Expect   168

    Goal Setting   170

    Seven Chakras & Associations • Illustration   172

32. RESOURCES

    Recommended Reading & Suggested Music   174

    The Healing Art of Conscious Breathing CD User's Guide—John Meneghini   176

    E3Live: *Earth's First Food*—Michael Saiber   178

    Zap-A-Kramp: *Nature's Solution to Cramping & Tetany*—Carlton Newman   182

    NaturalLifeNews.com   183

    Natural Life News & Directory   184

Introduction
to the Third Edition · 2019

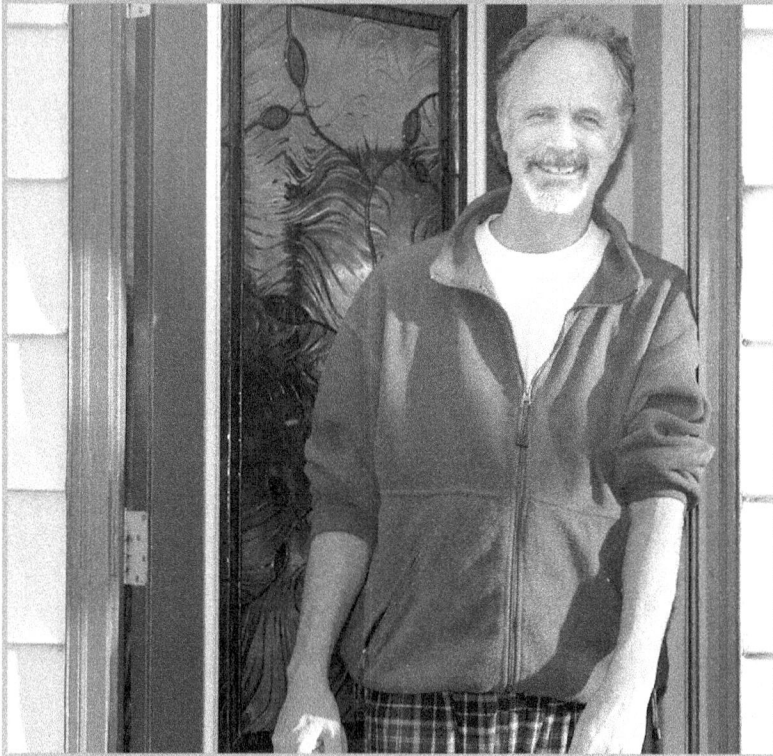

Well, it's 2019 and I'm 67 years old! This book, a multifaceted compilation of wisdom on natural healing—only a minor portion of which comes directly from me—all began when Debra Klein, a mystical lady, dropped some audiocassettes in my lap in 1979. I was in my late 20s and in my fourth year in the Navy in San Diego. I had fallen in with a band of friends interested in healing and spirituality.

I transcribed and edited those tapes, which grew in scope and number as we went along. That's Part Two of this book, first published alone in 1982 under the title, *Rebirthing According to Spirit—Healing through Breath, Light, Sound and Water*. I found myself among the pioneers of a practice called "rebirthing," which has since become known as "breathwork" in its many permutations. This original book ended up placing its stamp as foundational teachings on natural health, and I believe it stands on its own still today.

I moved on to other things in my life and career, including starting a family, and in about 2002, I got the prompting to take up breathwork again. As I collected new information and started to develop a half-day seminar, I got the idea to put this original work together with everything new I was learning and sharing with others. Thus was born this new book, with an adjusted title, and a host of new research and contributors. The second 2006 edition was mostly my seminar workbook, and since then I've gone through all 1000 of the copies printed.

Now, I suppose I'm preparing this (and myself) for posterity. I am adding a few key chapters and stories, getting the ISBN and bar code, and getting it up on Amazon and on my website, NaturalLifeNews.com. My Integral Breathwork Seminar is presented in Part Three in its entirety. I'm giving it all away for everyone to adapt, use, teach and experience in their own ways. I have taught this seminar more than 100 times and I'm still doing so, but now it's yours.

I still firmly believe that natural-healing methods must continue to re-emerge as our civilization learns from its mistakes and re-adopts more healthy ways of thinking and being that are more in harmony with God and with nature, from which She fashioned our bodies and through which Her Spirit flows.

Don't be too alarmed if this doesn't seem like much of a book at all, but more like a *hodge-podge!* Yes, I change the subject and even the authors quite a lot. But enjoy the variety and watch where it's leading you into the paradigm shifts of the ages.

Let's start this third (and final) edition off with a story and see where that leads us.

The Robust Boy

"Linda," a mother in her late thirties, attended one of my Integral Breathwork Seminars and had a good experience. A few months later she called and asked for a private session for her 16-year-old son who was experiencing bouts of asthma and allergies. I said sure, and invited her to attend the session—always a good idea with kids at that age. I was expecting a sickly boy but in walked "Sam," a rather robust teenager, dark hair, short and stout, with the body of a rugby player, well into puberty, and quite sure of himself.

Breathwork was all new to him and we started with some assessments. He was in great health overall, and his breathing was just fine, so I was a bit puzzled, but we proceeded. Not very long into his breathing session, maybe 10 minutes in, he sat up with a start, tears started running down his face and he said, "I couldn't breathe! I never want to feel THAT again!"

After settling him back down and using the breath to get him relaxed, on a hunch, I asked his mother, "Did Sam ever have a near-drowning experience?" She said, "Yes! When he was about a year old, we were at a park with a small brook run-

ning through it. I looked away for a second, and when I looked back, there he was face down under the water. We ran right up to him, got him breathing, and then had him checked out at the hospital. All seemed fine, and I had actually forgotten about that until you asked me."

We tried some more breathwork, but the session was really over after that experience and that revelation. It was really an unraveling of that experience from his memory banks. and sometimes, just having that "now I understand" moment is enough. One of the inner thoughts that, I would say, was playing out as a recording in Sam's brain (in the amygdala, to be exact), was exactly what he said when it came to the surface, "I never want to feel THAT again!" This is the typical recording that gets imprinted on the amygdala when any bad experience occurs, especially in the earliest years. Just like the toddler putting his hand on a hot stove, the brain learns NOT to do that again. But in Sam's case, in my view, what it set up was a tug of war with himself, blocking him from all the formative urges to explore, to grow, to be rambunctious, and replacing it with that scary memory of a near-death experience. Thus the allergies and the asthma, which is a way that the subconscious can hold someone back in the fear and reluctance aspects of "fight or flight."

That cycle of sabotage was broken for Sam, just by bringing that memory to the surface. Especially for a robust teenager, I believe that was all it took for him to jump off the massage table and be on to the next adventure.

At that age, you don't do much reflection, you don't often even say 'thank you.' "His mother and I did talk a few days later, and she said he was joking and rough-

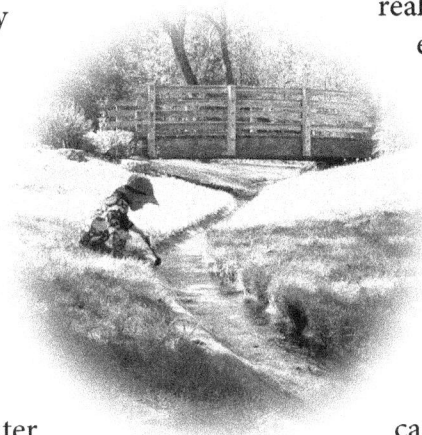

housing with his younger brother that afternoon, which was new behavior for him, so that's a sign that we was moving on. On his way home, he had a few things to say to his mother. One was, "Now there's ANOTHER thing wrong with me!" I stressed to Linda that, no, this was the ORIGINAL thing wrong with him and it's now resolved and unraveled from his subconscious, so he can make new choices, his immune system will immediately be less compromised, much stronger, so soon it will probably be goodbye to the asthma and the allergies.

At the tail end of our session, one of my daughters walked by, then 18 and quite attractive, apparently to Sam, walked by passing right between me and him on the massage table, and his mother. This seemed a bit odd to me, but that was the way to get downstairs to her room. Sam mentioned this to his mother, too, saying, "I'd go back there just to see HER again!" So apparently, Sam's libido was in good working order!

"Getting the War Out"

I have published the bi-monthly, regional magazine, *Natural Life News,* for over 16 years now. In 2007, I wrote an important article titled "Getting the War Out," now included in this book. In it, I refer to the groundbreaking therapy of Peter A. Levine, Ph.D., Somatic Experiencing®, which he uses for releasing stored trauma and PTSD. While my article was for soldiers in particular, the therapies described there apply to all trauma victims in general.

The Privilege of Fatherhood

As I pen this on Father's Day, I trust the readers will indulge me for a little fatherly bragging. There is no father who is not proud of his daughters, in this case, my twins, Vicky and Shelly. Here is Shelly's talent at skateboard art, which fetched a good price at the recent auction for Livingston's new skate park.

And here is a poem by Vicky, at 19 already a writer. Both will

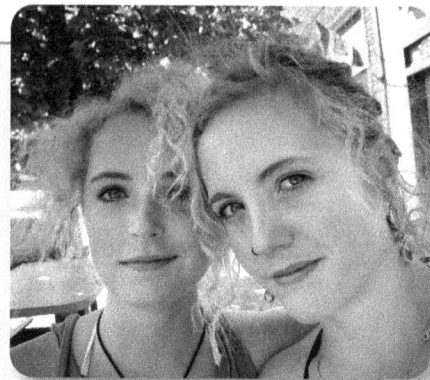

Vicky & Shelly Ouellette

be leaving soon to attend Prescott College, a progressive liberal-arts school in Arizona.

—*Denis O.*

Lightness

In my next life, I want to be
the wind on a hot, sticky day—
the sweet cool that caresses your warmth.
I want to be the stretch of a shadow—
the silhouette of a palm leaf
as it grows across the red dirt,
reaching, reaching...

I want to be the spray of a waterfall,
saying yes! I am something thunderous
and powerful but I will still
touch you gently.

I want to be a sprig of green shooting up
through a sidewalk crack, witness
to private acts of kindness, privy
to secret thoughts of self-destruction.
People will look at me and say,
"It's a miracle" and I will laugh because
they don't realize it is they
who are the miracle.

I want to be something untouchable.
The first break of dawn
as it splits through the dark
and lands on an unsuspecting scowl.
Seeping my warmth
into the broken places,
filling even the deepest fractures
with a liquid softness that grows
and swells and washes over you
in a way that you can't shake
the lightness in your soul for a full day.

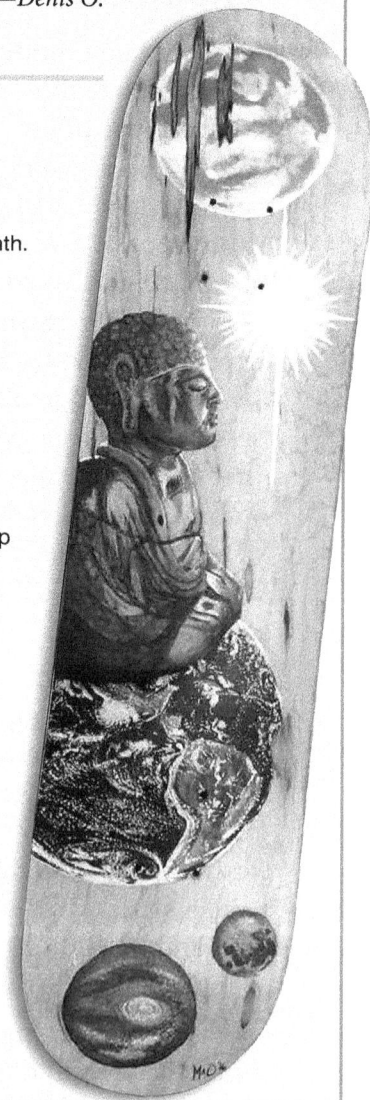

Natural Life News & Directory • July–August 2016

The methods Levine developed are wonderfully effective, as is breathwork, when done carefully and safely. In addition, Emotional Freedom Techniques (EFT), and Rapid Eye Technology (RET) and its cousin, Eye Movement Desensitization and Reprocessing (EMDR), as well as Psych-K, and Systemic Family Constellations—all of which are described in this article—have proven effective for PTSD.

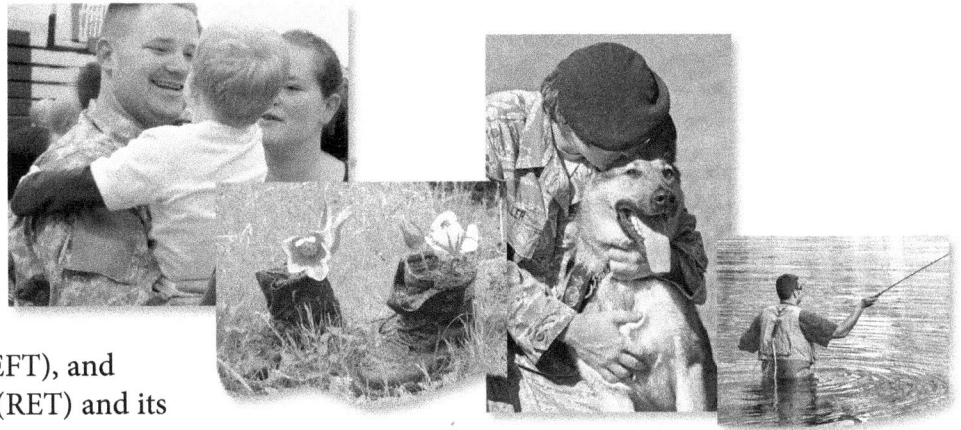

If the reader is interested in trauma release work, this lengthy article is a good place to start, as is a contribution by the Swiss psychotherapist Joy Manné, titled "Nothing as Powerful as Gentleness," also in this book. This type of work is sorely needed all over the planet. It is a major reason why I have pursued breathwork and bodywork as my life's calling. (Please note that in republishing "Getting the War Out," I have left all the contributors' advertisements intact, to show their faces and their credentials, but I can't vouch for their contact information, now 12 years later. You can always Google or Facebook them!)

It's always a wonder to me how readily our body's systems will right themselves, purge themselves, and return to homeostasis and health when given just a small amount of the right opportunity and coaxing, as depicted in Sam's case, above. For a child, small traumas are resolved with a good cry and a mother's hug. Most of us don't get through life without plenty of larger traumatic experiences—it's a rough-scrabble world, with a lot of abuse going around, in some cases built into our ancestry. It's up to the healers among us to help those in need.

John Upledger's life work also comes to mind, not only his wonderful CranioSacral Therapy®, but its offshoot, which he uncovered when releasing and discharging was happening spontaneously, called SomatoEmotional Release®. In his language, blockages caused by trauma, "energy cysts," can be dissipated, thus ridding the body of the need for adaptation and discomfort. All it takes for these releases to occur is a light touch and an attitude shift.

Similarly, there's the grassroots movement known as Re-evaluation Counseling, which I was involved with for years. All it takes there is some honest listening, and a verbal contradicting of a stubborn but erroneous self-concept to start the discharging and resolving of a long-held burden.

The Spiritual "Control"

As you move into Part Two (the channeled material) of this book, you will encounter discourses from three pairs of two spiritual beings, who on several occasions, instructed us on these topics of breathwork and natural healing. As I sat there transcribing these audiocassette recordings—this was in the late 1970s, mind you, before the days of computers—it struck me that these pairs consisted of one higher spiritual being and one who was much closer to the earth in terms of evolution and placement on the rungs of hierarchy, almost as if the higher being needed an intermediary, as a relay station, for this communication with earthlings to occur.

Mother Mary is lent assistance by Cochise, the Apache Chief. She brings blessings, while he delivers practical teachings and insights from the Akashic Records. In the second set, the arcane teachings of John the Divine are counterposed with the humorous and down-to-earth (astrally speaking) instructions of Tom McPherson. And again, the third set was John the Baptist with his fiery sermon, counterbalanced by Katherine the Healer (of unknown identity other than her name), whose valuable and practical teachings on energy healing I have used throughout my life's work.

I found an explanation for this pairing up in an article published by J. Douglas Kenyon, a friend and associate, in his *Atlantis Rising* magazine, from here in Livingston, Montana. The article is by Michael Tymn and titled, "The Case of Cora Scott Richmond—Nearly Two Centuries Later, Her Story Still Arouses Debate." (*AR #132*, Nov–Dec 2018) She was another astounding medium in the early days of such explorations. According to Harrison Barrett, her biographer, Cora was one of the most famous women in the world during the late 1800s. His 1895 biography of her is titled, *The Life Work of Cora L. V. Richmond*, and it describes how this phenomenon of a "spiritual control" works:

Some of the spirit communication came through in foreign languages, occasionally an ancient language, but a spirit named

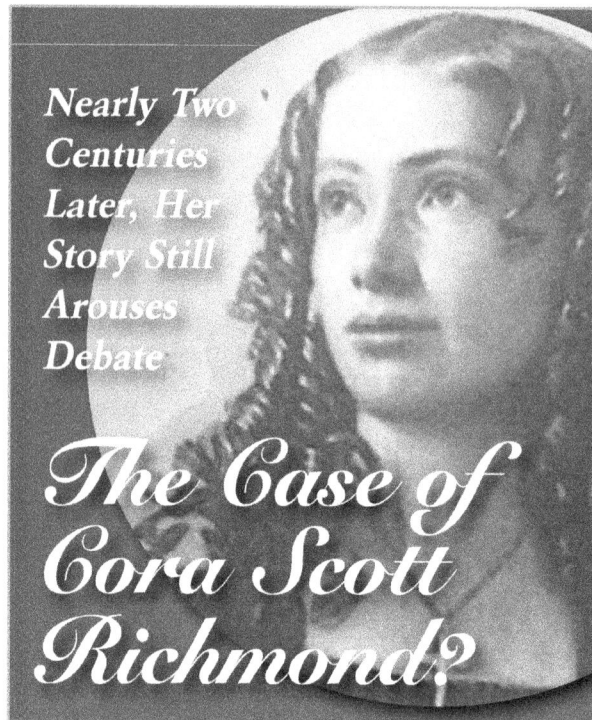

Nearly Two Centuries Later, Her Story Still Arouses Debate

The Case of Cora Scott Richmond?

Ouina, said to be an American Indian who had lived some 420 years earlier, served as Cora's chief guide and control, and was somehow able to interpret the foreign languages. Ouina also served as an intermediary for much more advanced spirits, who were at too great a vibration to effectively use Cora's organism.

I believe the sessions recorded in Part Two of this book, from my young-adult years in San Diego, with their specific teachings on natural healing and breathwork, came together because we, as a band of holistic healers with open minds and hearts, were ready to receive these truths. We were not daunted by the source from which this knowledge came. We felt no compunctions because we knew, loved, and trusted the mediums and the process. As the New Testament says, we did "test the spirits as to whether they are of God" (1 John 4:1), we did "discern" the messages (1 Cor. 12:10), and we did "hold on to what is good" (1 Thes. 5:21).

The Essene Gospel of Peace

As a young man, I devoured Edgar Cayce's works as the Sleeping Prophet. What he spoke of correlates well with Cochise's discourses from the Akashic Records on the healing temples of Atlantis outlined here. In addition, the teachings set down in 1981 in *The Essene Gospel of Peace*—apocryphal teachings of Jesus trans-

Your Inner Healer looks like you, speaks like you, feels as you do.
Your Inner Healer knows exactly your needs.

Breath is the rainbow bridge,
The rainbow bridge to your Inner Healer

Your Inner Healer doesn't care about technique.
Your Inner Healer simply waits in loving innocence
For the untainted truth carried on your Breath.

Your Inner Healer doesn't care about the "shoulds."
Your Inner Healer simply waits in loving innocence
To send with the Messenger of Breath
Whispers of truth to your Soul.

Breathworker Steve Moesong • Rhinelander, WI • Moesong.com

lated and edited by Edmond Bordeaux Szekely from the original Hebrew and Aramaic texts found in the Vatican Library—are a perfect correlation to the themes in this book.

As the stories are told there, Jesus asks those who have come to him for healing to fast and pray, and to embrace the natural elements in order to make their bodies clean and whole again. This is what he says about the angels of air, followed by the same exhortations to the angels of water and of sunlight (fire):

"Seek the fresh air of the forest and of the fields, and there in the midst of them shall you find the angel of air. Put off your shoes and your clothing and suffer the angel of air to embrace all your body. Then breathe long and deeply, that the angel of air may be brought within you. I tell you truly, the angel of air shall cast out of your body all uncleannesses that has defiled it without and within... No man may come before the face of God, whom the angel of air lets not pass. Truly, all must be born again by air and by truth, for your body breathes the air of the Earthly Mother, and your spirit breathes the truth of the Heavenly Father."

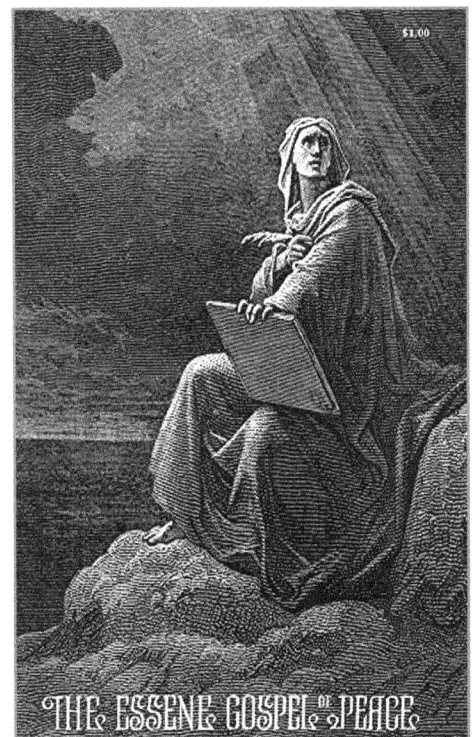

THE ESSENE GOSPEL OF PEACE

Omraam's Daily Meditations

Omraam Mikhaël Aïvanhov (1900–1986) was a Bulgarian philosopher, alchemist, mystic, and astrologer and a leading 20th-century teacher of Western Esotericism in Europe. As I read his biography and his Daily Meditations (available through Prosveta.com), so astounded was I at the alignment of his teachings with everything that this book stands for that I contacted the current president of his organization, who said it seems we were kindred spirits. He gave me permission to use twelve of those brief meditations in this book. (My only problem was that I have set aside many dozens of his quotes over the years!) Nine of them follow.

In the foreword to Omraam's biography, *The Mystery of Light,* Dr. Larry Dossey wrote, "One of the most striking qualities of Aïvanhov's teaching is the simplicity and clarity that shines through at every moment. What a joy to rediscover that authentic wisdom need not be opaque and impenetrable." Omraam speaks of healing yourself through nature's elements, in great part through the fire element in sunrise meditations, but also through air and water, and the "quintessence" that flows through all of nature. Some call this the Holy Spirit.

Omraam's methods of attaining physical and spiritual health often involve sunbathing or sungazing, and he named his system Solar Yoga. He freely acknowledged that the roots of his solar practices lay in ancient traditions he had learned from surviving masters from the Caucasian mountains, his homeland, and even from Tibet and India.

"Through my teaching," he said, "I want to impart to you some essential notions of the human being: how he is designed, his relationships with nature, and the exchanges he must make with the universe, if he is to drink from the springs of divine life." This is why Omraam, among all spiritual teachers, finds his way into

Omraam Mikhaël Aïvanhov

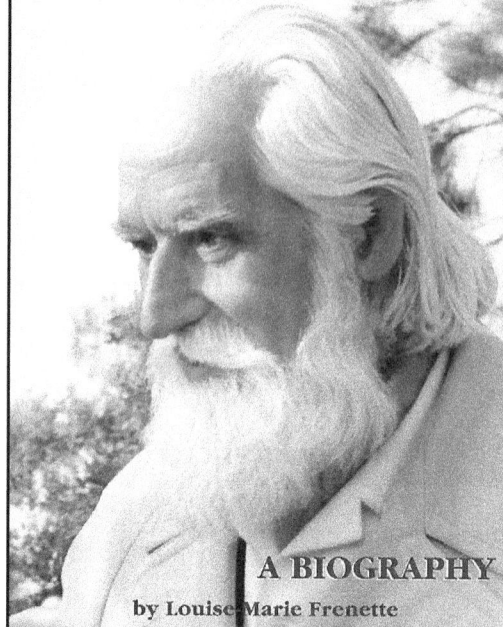

A BIOGRAPHY
by Louise-Marie Frenette

my 2019 introduction. Here are a few samples of his teachings that illustrate perfectly the themes I've attempted to collect and put forth in this book:

PRANA

At the beginning of creation God said, "Let there be light!' and from this light he made universal matter. Every morning at sunrise, we have an opportunity to intensify this living light within us, thanks to the "prana' contained in the air. Prana is an energy that exists throughout nature, in the earth, in water, air and fire, but it is mainly carried by the sun's rays, and through respiration we are able to capture it and introduce it into ourselves. Each particle of this prana is like a drop of crystalline water, a tiny, suspended sphere, filled with light. While we are concentrating on the sun, we absorb some of these spheres, these subtle particles, through our breathing, and in this way we strengthen not only our physical body but also our psychic organism. (4/13/08)

ELEMENTALS

For creation to become eloquent, alive and meaningful for you, you have to learn its language. Your whole life must be directed to this goal: to enter into communication with nature and its inhabitants. The inhabitants are everywhere: in the water, in the air, on the earth, in fire, in the mountains and trees, in the sun and the stars everywhere! And they greet us and give us signs. But who sees them? And who, also, sees nature as a luminous substance traversed by rays, whose colors and beauty no language can describe? If you wish these inhabitants to accept, help and support you, prepare yourself for entry into this immense world by giving it your attention, understanding and love. You already live in this world, you walk in it, but you must open your awareness still more to it and lift the veil that prevents you from seeing it. (9/22/08)

THE HIERARCHY OF NATURE

The different kingdoms of nature, along with the creatures that inhabit them, are interconnected. Whether or not we are aware of it, the beings both below and above us are connected to us. There is a living hierarchy in nature, and this link that connects us to all higher beings makes it possible for us to elevate ourselves. But we are also linked to all the beings below us—animals, plants and stones—and this link is extremely powerful. If our thoughts, feelings and actions are honest and pure, we receive beneficial forces from heaven, which pour into us through this continuous, living chain of creatures. But the divine currents do not stop at us; they pass through us and descend to the creatures below us in the animal, vegetable and mineral kingdoms, creatures that are also connected to us. In this way, each harmonious state we experience has a positive influence not only on the people around us but on the animals, plants and stones, which are also our brothers and sisters. (10/23/11)

RELATIONSHIP TO THE SUN

Everything on earth is transient, ephemeral, but above our heads the sun remains, unchanging and eternal, and that is where we must direct our gaze. When you seek the truth you must turn to something that doesn't pass away, that doesn't change. But it seems difficult for humans to find the right attitude towards the sun: Either they neglect it or they exaggerate its role; either they think it has nothing to do with religion or they worship it as an idol. They are mistaken in both cases. By giving the sun no place in their inner life, they are depriving themselves of an essential element. But to focus on the physical sun as though it were an idol is to regress to the mentality of those primitive peoples who worshipped the forces of nature. The sun must simply be a way of finding God, our inner sun. Each day, by contemplating it, by exposing ourselves to its rays and identifying with it, we increase our divine light, warmth and life. (5/19/08)

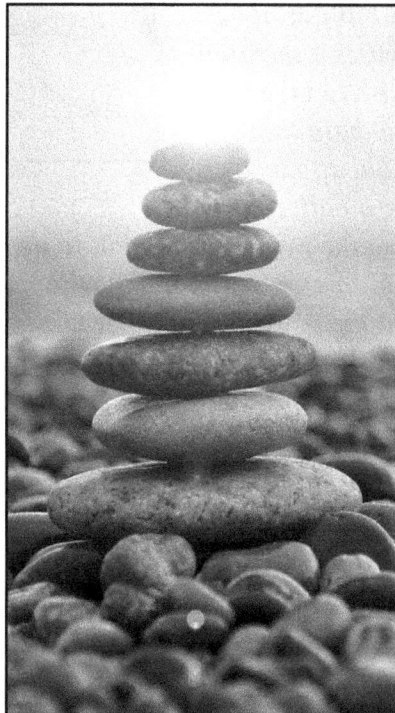

BREATH & FIRE

To breathe is to live. But life is neither to be confused with the act of breathing nor with air itself. Life has its origins in an element much subtler than air and for which air is a food: fire. Yes, life is found in a much higher realm, in fire. Air serves only to feed this fire, and without the presence of air the fire goes out. The lungs merely feed the fire that burns in the heart. The primary cause of life, therefore, is fire; and air, its brother, nourishes it. When man breathes his last, the fire goes out; when he exhales for the last time, life is extinguished. Since it is air that sustains the fire of life, we must pay great attention to the process of respiration. Do not imagine that just because you breathe, everything is fine. No, in most people, even though they are alive and breathing, this process has become weak, compromised. This is why they must make the effort to work with the breath so as to animate, purify, and intensify the life within them. (01/17/17)

BATHING IN WATER

Our everyday life is made up of numerous activities we consider prosaic, but it is always possible to give these prosaic activities a spiritual dimension. For example, if you wish to take a bath, why make do with a physical bath that will only get rid of a bit of dirt? It should also be a bath that washes you on all levels, a bath that purifies you. So, before you get into the water, speak to it, to the entities that live in it, and say to them, 'You creatures who live in this water, I am happy to make contact with you today, because I know God has given you the power to rid my whole being of impurities. That is why I'm speaking to you, so you can work on me." And you touch the water, you bless it and invoke the power God has over water, the light of God and the purity of God. When you speak to water in this way, as to a very precious element in which creatures of great purity live, you are already entering into contact with it on other planes, and when you begin to wash yourself, you also reach your etheric, astral and mental bodies. You feel relieved of all the psychic impurities you have accumulated, and after your bath you are ready to get back to work with renewed strength. (08/14/09)

PURPOSE OF INCARNATION

What are we doing on earth? What is our purpose in coming here? We have come to earth for a very important reason: to study matter and work with the forces, which animate it. We are spirits who have been given bodies so that we can function in the world of matter. Some think the Lord has designed things very badly: since man is a spirit, instead of incarnating in a body that restricts and imprisons him, he should have remained in the spirit world, in the light and magnificence of heaven. No, in his great wisdom the Lord decided otherwise, and contrary to appearances our descent into matter does not exile us far from him, for matter is of the same essence as God. It is a condensation of the divine force. (12/6/18)

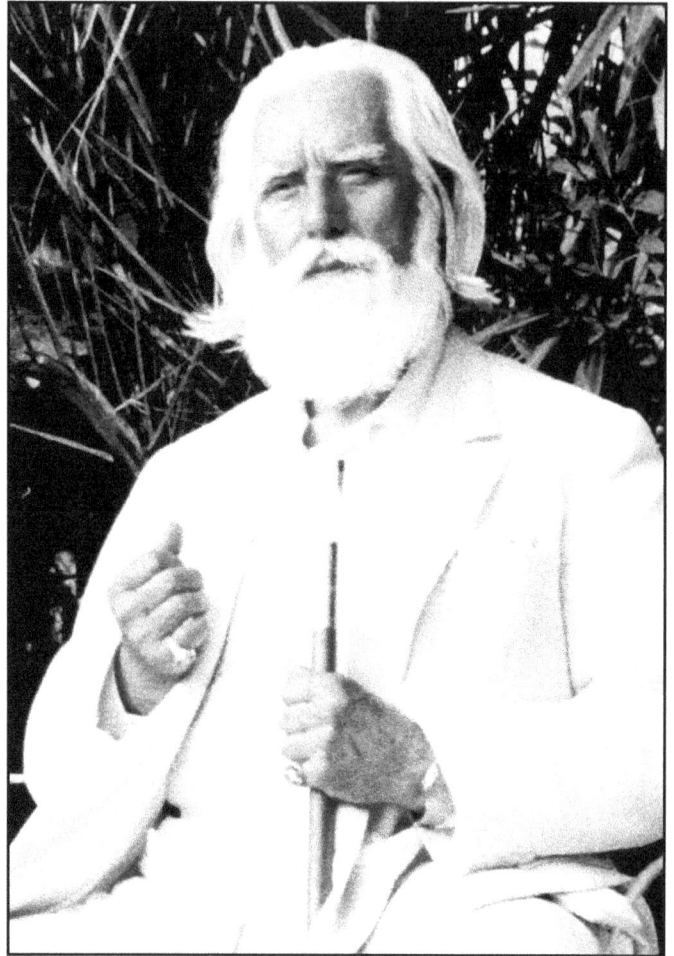

PUTTING LIGHT FIRST

You must put light in first place. For light is present in all things. When you become imbued with this truth, your whole life will be transformed. If, when you eat, you are conscious that your food—fruit, vegetables—is a condensation of the solar rays it has received, you create better physiological conditions for these rays to be absorbed and distributed throughout your organism. If you breathe with the conviction that you can attract light into yourself through your breathing, you are preparing yourself to receive celestial light, the spirit of God. For the light you see, the light coming from the sun, is only the most material form of light. Behind this light there are other, subtler lights, and if you know how to relate to these, how to nourish yourself with them, they will bring you eternal life. (03/23/09)

THE POWER OF MUSIC

Angelic beings appreciate harmony and are attracted by music and singing. This is a belief that goes back to very ancient times. However far back we go in human history, sacred ceremonies have been accompanied by music and singing. Celestial beings love music; they themselves are music, which is why so many artists have depicted paradise filled with angels singing and playing all kinds of instruments. Sounds, whether instrumental or vocal, have enormous power, not only because they can be pleasing to the ear, but also because the vibrations they produce are so strong. We must, therefore, become aware of the power of music and find out how we can use its vibrations, which when amplified by the feelings of those who are playing or listening, create a conducive atmosphere for beings of light to visit us. (03/20/11)

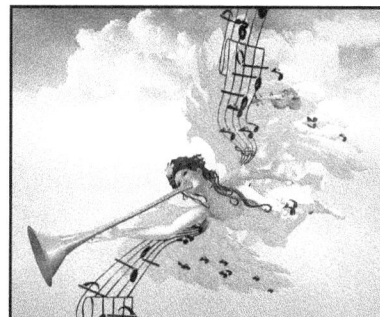

So Grateful!

My life has been blessed with so many experiences, teachers, and healings. Along with the breathwork seminars, I've been in a bodywork practice, off and on, for all these years too. I tried to count how many massages I've done and it's now over 15,000. As an NCBTMB Approved Provider, I have taught other bodyworkers how to incorporate more breathing work into their sessions. (I've included an article on bodywork toward the end of the book, as I pass the torch and hang up my oil holster, one of these years...)

Grateful am I for all the friendships I've made with so many of the world's most wonderful therapists and healers, some in person and still more by absorbing and assimilating their work into my own. Grateful I am for all the clients I've been able to help. When you get someone out of stress, you change their decision-making and therefore, the course of their lives. This is a privilege that truly humbles me.

May YOU find inspiration here that fits with your soul and mind and your direction in life. May you look deeper into the invisible worlds that surround you, and through your therapy and spiritual practice, may you open your perceptions to those worlds and the loving beings that inhabit them, both in nature and in higher realms. All you have to do is stay positive, and share love and light, and they will rally around you—even the tiniest electrons of the Holy Spirit will gather around you like moths to a flame.

As you bless life on earth, all is lifted along with you. Thank you for reading and the sharing what you've learned and become.

— Denis Ouellette • April 2019

*Special
Acknowledgment
for the Contributions of:*

Michael Grant White
Debra Klein
Kevin Ryerson
Michael Richard
J. Michael Wood
Sol Luckman
John C. Ledbetter
Paul von Boeckmann
Daniel P. Reid
Leon Chaitow
Thomas Goode
Dan Brulé
Joy Manné
John Meneghini
Michael Saiber

& to all those who
contributed sidebars
and personal stories

❧—❧ ❧—❧ ❧—❧

Gratitude to the Editors:

Olivia Hoyt
Joan Nemeth
Linda Locke

PART ONE
Inhale!

Y ou can tap into the healing powers already within your body and make use of nature's purest and simplest elements to do so. You can use breath, light, sound, and water to return to your innate wholeness, beyond what you even thought possible. The subtle life forces flowing through these elements are called *pranas* in the ancient Sanskrit. We absorb and use these pranas constantly. Of earth's life-giving elements, air is the most precious. Oxygen is abundant in the air, in water, and in chlorophyll-bearing vegetation. Subtler still are the pranas contained in light, both sunlight and artificial, and in the vibrations of pure sound and high-quality music. The material that follows explains how to access the powerful yet little-appreciated healing properties within these elements.

This book also contains information on ancient healing practices that came into my possession over 25 years ago. At that time I published this material and incorporated it into my holistic-health and breathwork practice. Over the years, I have combined this ancient knowledge with present-day science in a system I call Integral Breathwork". The information is compiled here for your use. We invite you to experience its healing power at one of our Integral Breathwork seminars. We start with the breath as a healing tool, because breath is basic and immediate. It works especially well for people new to alternative therapies. This book is a manual on the practice of breathwork, incorporating its use with light, sound, and water. We use the breath first to clear away toxins and reawaken the senses. Once this foundation is laid and some skill is achieved, we can better perceive and work with the more subtle of the elements and energy forces.

Your breath can be your best friend! It is ever present, providing you with life-giving oxygen and subtle energy from birth until death. It supports you by working heavily in times of exertion and stress and by calming you with slower, gentler patterns when it's time to rest and repair. Can a mother giving birth have any better ally than her breath? The breath is automatic—it works unconsciously, like your beating heart and immune system, your digestion and elimination. It is a pivotal function of the autonomic nervous system. When we bring the breath under our conscious control for healing, it opens up a whole new world. By using the breath in specific and powerful ways, it becomes a doorway into the hallowed inner workings of our physical body, our cellular memories, and our subconscious mind. Through cellular oxygenation (inhale) and the release of toxins along with carbon dioxide (exhale), and by skillfully directing the healing pranas of life, we can maintain and repair not only the respiratory system but *all* of our internal systems. When some of this homework is done, we can begin to use the breath as a vehicle for deepening consciousness and apprehending our higher purpose in life.

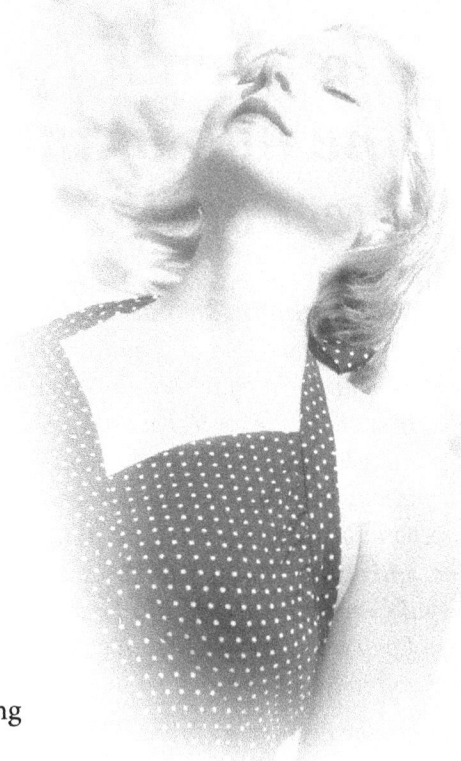

"The breath is at the hub of the wheel of life."

Use the breath as your pivotal tool for branching out in all directions for healing and rejuvenation. When invited in with a little vigor, both oxygen and energy will penetrate the physical, mental, and emotional parts of yourself. The body will respond by relieving stress, expelling toxins, and opening energy blockages. When these pathways become clear, the breath can lead you into an awareness of its connection to All of Life.

Since the beginning of recorded history, the breath and other natural elements have been used for healing. Breathwork will enhance and multiply the benefits of any healing modality you are practicing. Those receiving bodywork who breathe fully during their session can double the benefits of their therapy. Yoga and Pilates, hydrotherapy, nutritional and herbal cleanses, and spiritual practices all blend wonderfully with the clearing power of the breath. Bodyworkers and therapists who breathe fully will be more effective and remain energized and well-balanced.

We start with a scientific understanding and experience of what optimal breathing is. Then we partake in a breathwork session to reap the benefits of full-body oxygenation and detoxification. This session has predictable and cyclical phases and will gently clear away one layer of debris at a time. You can set specific goals for your healing, yet you remain open, trusting in the body's innate healing mechanisms to take you reliably on the safest path toward wholeness.

We all store tension in our muscles. But why? Science is advancing in its understanding of the link between body and mind. We're learning that the muscular tissues and the cells themselves have a subconscious memory. Often long after a physical injury or emotional trauma has passed, its shadow can linger on as tension, chronic pain, disability, and self-protectiveness. Emotional reactions, behavioral patterns, and negative mental attitudes can become imprinted and seem difficult to clear away. The breath is a remarkably effective way of getting in there to unlock and release these imprints.

Many of us have a breath that is shallow or nearly shut down. Many of us don't breathe diaphragmatically. This can be both a cause and effect of illness, injury, or the disabling of other internal, automatic systems. **We will always breathe enough to survive, but can our breath—and our life—be fuller?** Can our internal engines work more optimally? Take a moment to notice how you are breathing right now. If you are not breathing as freely as you would like, it could be of great value for you to pursue breathwork.

A big, beautiful breath should be like an ocean wave. On the inhale, as the lungs fill and the diaphragm descends, you should feel a 360° expansion in your lower torso. [See *The Pear, the Cone & the Wave* in Appendix.] This momentum builds and rises with a steady determination to its peak as air fills the rib cage and chest areas. The spine ripples as the wave moves up your body. The muscles of the neck and shoulders should remain relaxed, rather than bulging to lift the ribs off the lungs, as high-chest breathers often do. Then, without holding at the top, we exhale. The momentum spills over and crashes to the shore as we relax and release totally. This kind of exhale even sounds like a crashing ocean wave. We may find ourselves resting before the natural reflex prompts us to take in another breath.

Breathwork is fun and provides instant gratification. Take a few minutes right now to try the following rhythmic breathing technique. Sit or lie down comfortably somewhere. It's even better if you can be in the fresh air. Close your eyes. Relax and start focusing on your breath. As you breathe in through your nose, first fill your lower lungs. As your diaphragm descends, feel the expansion in your abdomen and sides and even in your lower back and kidney areas. Then feel your ribs open sideways (not upwards) as you fill your middle and upper lungs. Finally, feel your chest rising a bit.

Now fill your head with air. (Humor me on this one.) Traveling along with the physical breath is a corresponding energy flow, understood well by yogis, that you can experiment with. As you breathe in, the energy rises up your spinal column and along your *meridians* (energy pathways). The flow doesn't stop at the top of your lungs. When you get near the top of your inhale, breathe in a little more as you swing the energy around the back and over the top of your head. Feel the cycle coming to rest in the vicinity of your mouth and nose. Next, simply exhale, totally relaxing as you do.

Another helpful visualization is to imagine that oxygen and energy are going directly from your nasal cavities into your brain as you breathe in, refreshing and cleansing you mentally. Repeat the above process for twenty breaths or so. Now how do you feel? Probably refreshed, grounded, more calm, and centered in the present moment. Maybe you're thinking about how your breath really *is* your best friend.

Yes, you can benefit greatly by improving the quality and quantity of your breathing, and this book will show you how. Yes, breathing is automatic and unconscious, but through conscious breathing you can access your body's internal systems. **Would you drive your car without opening the hood for regular maintenance or repair?**

Let's take a closer look at your body's main fuel, oxygen. It is more necessary than food for keeping cells healthy and happy. Oxygen is like gold! It's your primary source of energy. Oxygen is free, but like gold, it can be elusive because most people breathe at about 20% of their full capacity. As a consequence, their cells suffer. The good digestion resulting from diaphragmatic movement and the good detoxing from an efficient exhale usually don't happen well. This leaves them fatigued and sick.

The brain and nervous system thrive on oxygen. Oxygen displaces harmful free radicals, neutralizes environmental toxins, and helps destroy infectious bacteria, parasites, microbes, and viruses. These invaders, along with cancer cells, are anaerobic, which means they cannot live in oxygen-rich environments.

Oxygen shortage has been linked to every major illness, including heart conditions, poor digestion and elimination, asthma and sinus problems, arthritis, yeast infections, sexual dysfunction, and auto-immune diseases. Some indicators of low-oxygen levels are fatigue, muscle aches, forgetfulness, heart palpitations, cold extremities from poor circulation, and excessive allergies or colds.

In 1930s, Otto Warburg won the Nobel Prize in Medicine *twice* for discovering that only oxygen-starved cells weaken, mutate, and become cancerous. Cells starved for oxygen become something else entirely. Warburg found that rather than living and breathing aerobically, oxygen-starved cells live from the fermentation of sugars, and all their normal functions die off *except for reproduction.*

The benefits of breathwork include increased longevity and vitality, cell regeneration, emotional and mental well-being, and trauma resolution. Our Integral Breathwork seminar is a combination of physiological breathing work and transformational breathwork. The word *integral* means "lacking nothing essential." We start by doing assessments and several exercises for improving breathing mechanics. Then we lie down for a gentle one-hour breathing session to experience full-body oxygenation and detoxing. Several of the seminar processes are outlined in the Appendix to this book.

Many of us are too often stuck in "fight or flight." Because of stress, poor diet, and oxygen depletion, the autonomic nervous system stays in emergency mode on the sympathetic side. After one breathwork session, most people will feel what it's like to have a nervous system that's finally at peace, free to focus on "rest, digest and heal" on the parasympathetic side. Your body knows just what to do with extra oxygen and how to cleanse itself when given the chance. It will respond by releasing stored toxins and tension and clearing out cellular memories. Every session will be uniquely suited to your body's most pressing needs.

For a glimpse at the power and potential of this work, let's start with a few stories from people who have used breathwork to great advantage in their own healing. Then we'll explore the autonomic nervous system in more detail to understand the fight-or-flight syndrome in ways that Western medicine is now only beginning to understand and embrace. Mike White of Breathing.com checks in next with a more detailed look at oxygen. Then we'll have some fun exploring the exhale.

Part Two presents the remarkable channeled materials I came upon and, in part, witnessed and then transcribed 25 years ago,* on the ancient origins of this healing modality, along with timeless instructions. While this book focuses primarily on breathwork, it also explores the healing energies inherent within light, sound, water, and earth. To discover how sound and light activate healing in the DNA, read Sol Luckman's article in Part Three. Next, John Ledbetter describes the power of the earth's and our body's own electric fields. Thanks to both Sol and John for their contributions, and thanks to all who have contributed sidebars for their added perspectives.

In Part Three, you'll find further tools, guidelines and more stories on the healing practice we call Integral Breathwork, which integrates physiological breathing work with transformational breathwork.

Life is a miracle. Yet some of life's most precious secrets are hidden in nature's simplest and purest of elements. It's time for you to discover them! ▨

❧——❧ ❧——❧ ❧——❧

*NOTE: If you are reading book this in its Third (and final) Edition, published in 2019, the 25 years mentioned above has become 40 years!

Releasing Vietnam

Dustin Fox, CAMT • Emigrant, MT

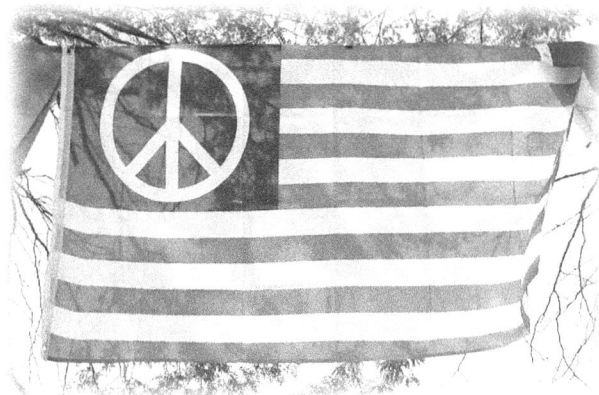

My name is Dustin and I am a Massage Therapist. My first exposure to breathwork was during a massage I was giving to Denis Ouellette. He was breathing differently than anyone I had ever massaged before. His inhales were deep, and his exhales were really full and completely emptied his lungs. I had never studied breathing techniques but was fascinated by this self-cleansing approach to breathing. I signed up to attend his next breathwork seminar. I noticed that several essential health issues were being addressed. As a therapist, I was fascinated by the facts presented as to how we actually breathe, compared to how we could breathe to facilitate better health and well-being.

During the next few months, I attended four breathwork seminars and felt better after each one. But there were deeper issues that I needed to address that had settled into my very soul. It was at my fifth seminar that I felt this would be the day to identify and release whatever it was that was holding me in such turmoil. Following the instructions and breath measurement exercises, we partnered with someone in an atmosphere of safety and honesty. We shared the issues that we wished to address during our breathwork session. I realized it was time to go after my remaining Post Traumatic Stress Syndrome from the Vietnam War, over 35 five years ago. These "cellular memories" were still holding me in a depressed state and draining me of my health and spiritual contentment. They needed to be released.

As we began to breathe, I felt a stiffness set in throughout my body. The cramping in my hands began to get a bit intense. Denis came over and assisted me through the process. As I allowed myself to relax and breathe through the memories of pain and trauma, they left me. It took one more session for this to be complete. At one point during that sixth one, Denis said he was concerned about me because I looked as gray as a ghost. I think death itself was leaving me! I now feel completely content and cleansed of that trauma and depression.

P.S. **BLOOD TESTS.** Last year, before I began breathwork, I was advised by my physician to get a blood test as part of my annual checkup. Under the microscope, I was surprised to see that my blood cells were not round, but clustered together and misshapen. I was advised that this causes a reduction in the ability of the circulatory system to do its job of delivering oxygen and nutrients to the body while removing waste products. This condition had an effect on my liver, kidney, brain and heart function. Healthy blood cells are supposed to float free within the system and are almost perfectly round. The doctor advised me to modify my diet to reduce sugar and fats, to exercise and most importantly, to improve my breathing to facilitate the reduction of stress and to increase my level of oxygen intake.

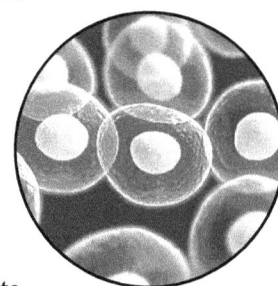

About ten months later, after five breathwork sessions and plenty of breathwork on my own, I returned for another blood test and was gratified to see that my sickly-looking, large blood-cell clusters were all but gone. The blood was rich with oxygen. Other tests showed that my organ function was within a normal range. I did make small changes in my diet and I do some light exercises, but doing the breathwork regularly is what brought my cells back to life!

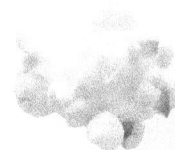

Popcorn on a Stove

Brenda Frye • Emigrant, MT

I've been told over the years that I was a shallow breather, but I was never instructed on how to change my breathing. My history of work in the medical community gave me the knowledge of how important oxygen is, but I figured—I was breathing, so what was the problem? I was invited by a friend to attend a breathwork seminar and I went out of curiosity. I have attended several of them now and each one has brought me to a different and higher level of awareness and self-healing.

One of these sessions stands out for me. We are asked to scan our bodies and to select areas that we wanted to focus the healing breath on. I had suffered a severe injury to my right ankle over a year previously and I was still experiencing discomfort. As I lay down to begin the breathing, I concentrated on the rhythm and depth of my breath. As time passed, my body began to tingle and then vibrate all the way down to my toes. Also it was during this time my ankle began to stiffen and became quite painful. At first I thought, "What is this? It hurts!" But then I remembered the instruction that, as our cells release the memory of a trauma, we may re-experience the original pain, so I kept my focus on my breathing. Slowly the pain subsided but my ankle still felt stiff. I began to move it in a slow rotation. I felt it cracking repeatedly! It sounded like popcorn on a stove. I soon recognized that my ankle was now moving with ease and without any pain at all. As I lay there contemplating with joy what had just happened, I realized that I had released my ankle's injury from my cells and had breathed new life into it.

It is now months later and the ankle is still pain-free. I continue to attend these seminars and do breathwork on my own. I'm always learning more about the benefits of proper rhythmic and full breathing. The Breath of Life is there for my joy and health! I am now happy to be learning how to share this gift with others.

Better Than Ten Therapy Sessions!

M.W. • Bozeman, MT

I first decided to attend a breathwork seminar because of problems I had with chronic fatigue syndrome, since I thought that increased oxygen to the body would help relieve my symptoms. I was in for a surprise when I found that during the session, I was able to experience and release childhood wounds, and specifically, issues of abandonment. I had not come prepared with a box of tissues nor had I expected that my eye makeup would be all gone before the session was over. At the end I thought, "Wow! This was better than ten therapy sessions!" During the next couple of sessions, in addition to increased oxygenation of the cells and body, which provided more clarity and greater well-being, I was able to release more past traumas.

During my latest session, I was in for another surprise. At first I started to fall asleep, but a facilitator came by to wake me up and told me that my drowsiness was due to toxins being released into my bloodstream. As I continued to breathe, the music that was playing reminded me of my search for my perfect love. I recalled the memories and emotions of loves found and lost in my life. I mourned these experiences and felt the emotion of separation from my perfect love. After feeling this, I came in touch with feelings of the pain of separation from God, my first love. After experiencing this loss, I moved into an unexpected, beautiful experience of my oneness with God. The closest I can come to describing this is as a feeling of total joy, love, and peace. I have been on the spiritual path for many years and have had other spiritual experiences, but this transcendental bliss was very nurturing to my soul.

I came to my first breathwork class with the naive intention of just healing my physical body, and I realized I was healing my emotional body. Now, after this last session, I know this work actually heals all our bodies—the physical, emotional, mental, and memory bodies. Thus breathwork is a vehicle for personal transformation. It was very meaningful for me to discover the benefits of this work for myself. I have found breathwork to be one of those hidden gems—much more than meets the eye! ▪

Asthma, Arterial Fibrillation & Rebounding

Marlenea La Shomb • Livingston, MT

I have been dealing with asthma since I was a child, and I have carefully avoided foods and situations that I know will trigger an attack. After my first breathwork seminar, I learned how to move out of the sympathetic side of my autonomic nervous system ("fight or flight") by controlling and directing my breath. Three days later, I was at a girlfriend's birthday party. There was dairy, a lot of cat hair, and smoking—three big asthma triggers for me. As I left, I felt a strong asthma attack coming on. During my drive home, I did the diaphragmatic breathing and slowed down on my exhale. I was able to avert the asthma attack within a half hour, where it would usually take me 4 to 5 hours of struggle, plus using an inhaler or drugs.

I also learned a method for calming an asthma attack by lying down and lifting one leg in the air, then slowly lowering my leg to the ground while exhaling and saying *"Sssshhhh!"*

A friend of mine also attended who has a problem with arterial fibrillation, where the valve between the upper and lower chambers of the heart will get stuck open, causing blood to drip back down, so the heart is unable to pump the blood properly. This causes light-headedness, nausea, and a racing heart. He becomes extremely weak and needs to get down on the ground with his head between his knees. The next day at a job site, he felt his heart racing again. He dropped his tool belt and got down on his knees. He used a technique he learned to calm his system and direct a slow exhale and energy to his heart area. As with asthma, the non-closing of this valve can be triggered by stress. He is now able to bring this condition into balance and get the valve to close every time just by controlling his breath. He once went to the emergency room when this happened, and they told him there was nothing they could do for him except use the electro-defibrillator to shock the valve into closing. We are glad he has a natural method, along with foot-zone balance and essential oils, to handle this problem.

I have since become a Naturopathic Doctor and certified reboundologist. I use breathwork in all of my work. Rebounding uses the natural forces of acceleration, deceleration and gravity to move all the fluids in the body and to bring oxygen to all the cells. It's like having a second set of lungs! ▪

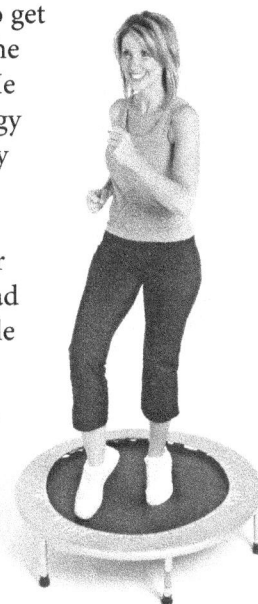

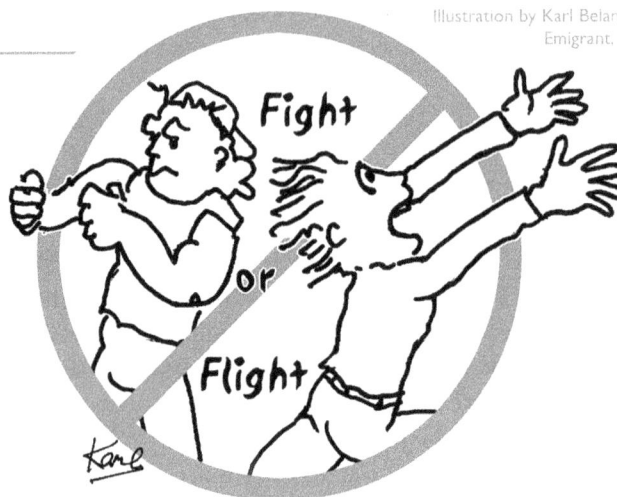

Illustration by Karl Belanger
Emigrant, MT

Are You Stuck in "Fight-or-Flight"?

Do you tend to see the glass as half empty? Do you find yourself dwelling on worries, fears, or resentments more than you'd like to? Do you overreact to stress or upset? When something bad happens, do you say, "I knew it!" rather than, "Well, OK, now what?" These are common emotional indicators of being stuck in fight-or-flight. This condition shows up in our bodies as an imbalance in the autonomic nervous system called overactive sympathetic tone. The good news is that it's adjustable.

Many people deal with this at a more severe level. They have anxiety or depression too often and can't shake a negative outlook. Their sex drive and general aliveness may be low. Those with this imbalance often develop high blood pressure, digestive disorders, peptic ulcers, poor circulation, or migraine headaches. The longer people stay stuck in it, the worse the symptoms can get. Chronic pain, anxiety attacks, fibromyalgia, and other stress-related or immune-deficiency diseases may develop. Western medicine has opted to treat the symptoms and has not always understood the cause. Treating high blood pressure with medications that block the beta receptors or treating ulcers with antacid pills can allay symptoms but can also create imbalances in other parts of the body.

It's common for people who are overanxious or out-of-sorts to eat too much. This can come from a subconscious desire to get some relief from fight-or-flight by forcing the activation of digestion, which cools down the nervous system and brings it to the parasympathetic side. [See diagram next page.] But there's a better way to do this!

Dr. Andrew Weil, a proponent of integrative and holistic medicine, points out that in the West, there isn't even a standardized diagnosis for this nervous-system imbalance, but practitioners of oriental medicine have known about it for centuries. What's the easiest, most natural way to bring your nervous system back into balance? It's through conscious breathing!

HERE'S HOW IT WORKS.

You have two nervous systems: the voluntary one (central nervous system) and the involuntary, automatic one (autonomic nervous system). The autonomic system governs all the unconscious functions of the body, such as heart rate, circulation, and blood pressure, hormone secretion, digestion, elimination, and sexual function. The disorders listed earlier are all imbalances in these internal, automatic systems. But how do we access the autonomic system if this part of us is hidden, unconscious, and automatic? How do we get in there to reestablish balance or to do maintenance and repair? Breathing is the doorway, because it's the only system in our bodies that works both consciously and unconsciously.

The autonomic system has two opposing sides—the sympathetic and the parasympathetic. These are the two sides of one gauge, one runs hot, so to speak, and one cold. Ideally they should interact freely with each other and come into dominance depending on the situation. We are meant to move into the sympathetic side in times of physical exertion, excitement, emergency, and stress. That's the hot side, and it serves a valuable purpose whenever fight-or-flight is necessary!

When the sympathetic system is stimulated, heart rate increases, as does sweating. The blood vessels dilate in the large muscle groups, so more blood is diverted to them. Adrenaline rushes and we are alert and prepared to handle whatever extra stress we are in. Brain dominance shifts from the frontal lobes to the posterior, from the ability to use complex logic and higher logic and intelligence, to using only black-and-white, yes-or-no, primitive decision making.

The problem is that many of us can't easily rebalance to a neutral or relaxed state when the stress or upset has passed. We are supposed to move from this hot reflex to periods of cooling down when the parasympathetic nerves and their functions take over. This usually occurs during sleep and with daily food digestion and waste elimination. The immune system and many other complex internal functions only perform well when the parasympathetic is active. When we're stuck in the sympathetic, the parasympathetic functions don't all get their chance. So how and why do we get stuck in the sympathetic and how do we get unstuck? Our current load of daily stress and constant overstimulation play their parts, as does poor nutrition. But unresolved past distress compounds it.

Here's a graphic example that we use in our breathwork seminars. Take an empty clear plastic drinking bottle, and squeeze and dent it all over. This illustrates the state of many people's nervous systems and of their breathing patterns. Every physical, mental, or emotional pain or trauma that we have endured throughout our lives, but which has not been properly released and healed, leaves its record as a dent in our nervous systems, and a self-protecting, self-defensive reflex memory gets stored in our physical cells. We call these cellular memories. Over time, as these memories build up, we lose functionality and flexibility in the damaged areas of our bodies. We may also become more negative and rigid mentally, and more fearful or angry emotionally, especially when something happens that reminds us of this trauma from the past. We are apt to overreact to our daily stresses because of those earlier similar memories we are still dealing with. We tend to feel less safe emotionally, which can lead to the self-defensive behavior patterns of fight (belligerence) or flight (withdrawal).

Soon a host of symptoms can start to appear. The major ones are listed. We are witnessing here the overlapping interplay between the physical,

the emotional, and the mental parts of ourselves and how damage can cross over. Addressing this holistically through the power of breathing can activate the healing process.

So back to our dented bottle. We blow into it and some of the dents will pop out. Blow again and more will come out. The bottle can eventually return to its original shape. In the body, we call that original form our *energetic blueprint*. Could it be that easy? Well, almost!

CONSCIOUS BREATHING HEALS!

The breath is the doorway to the healing of the imbalance in the autonomic nervous system and all the bodily functions it governs. When we use specific regenerative breathing techniques and engage in consciously expanding our shut-down or imbalanced breathing patterns, we are pushing against those dents—taking our bodies on a trip to the "body shop." We start the process of oxygenation and detoxification at a cellular level. This allows our bodies to clear away stored memories of distress and trauma. This can result in the balancing of the respiratory, nervous, and endocrine systems— in fact, all of our systems. It works and it feels great! Most people who come to our seminars feel more de-stressed and at peace than they've felt in a long time.

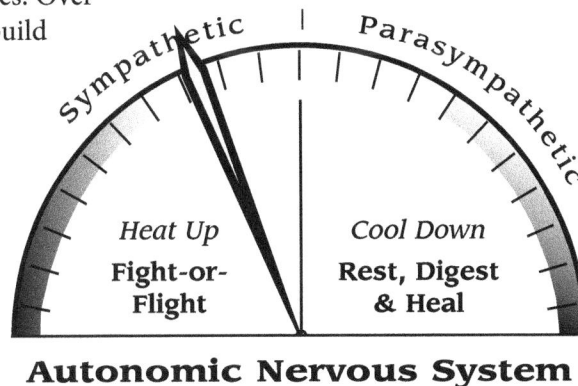

There are many methods we can use to naturally resolve the past and heal our bodies, our minds, and our emotions. People are catching on to the fact that suppression of symptoms through drugs, whether medical or recreational, is a lose/lose equation. This doesn't solve the core problem, and it often creates more problems of its own. Breathwork is a safe, fun, and natural alternative.

A BETTER SEX LIFE. Sex that is enjoyable and relaxed is only possible when that gauge governing the sympathetic and the parasympathetic is resting comfortably in the middle and free to toggle back and forth as needed. Working

Sympathetic | Parasympathetic

Heat Up
Fight-or-Flight

Cool Down
Rest, Digest & Heal

Autonomic Nervous System

simultaneously, both these systems are responsible for sexual arousal and orgasm. If the dial is too far off in one direction, either temporarily or chronically, you are either too stressed (over-amped) or too relaxed (disinterested) for sex.

"OK, I'M SOLD. SO WHAT DO I DO?"

Even slowing down and paying attention to your breath will advance you in the direction of a balanced nervous system. Find a time when you can sit down, preferably in fresh air, for some good breathing. Close your eyes and still yourself. For this cleansing type of breath, we do mouth breathing, although most normal breathing will be through the nose.

After a good exhalation, fill yourself with air starting with the lower abdomen. Allow the sides and lower back to expand also. After you are nice and full down below, let your ribs expand outward, but try not to lift your ribs upward with your shoulder and neck muscles. Don't hold your breath at the top. Just let it go freely and easily—like a wave crashing on the shore and spilling the momentum it has gathered. Your breath and your spine will make such a wave as you breathe this way. Feel your body relaxing totally on the exhale. No need to push out with force or purse the lips and blow with a *"Whoooo"* sound. The sound should be *"Haaaaww"* passing through an open throat and a relaxed jaw. If it feels natural, allow yourself to pause at the bottom of the exhale. As you empty your lungs, relax; then the vacuum will be filled again with the next in-breath.

If you are stressed, agitated, or upset (over-active sympathetic) you can modify this full breathing technique to calm down and get back into balance by simply slowing down on the exhale. Breathe in for a count of four and breathe out for a count of eight. Keep it gentle, deep, rhythmic and smooth, with no pauses at the top or bottom of the breath. You can do ten or twenty breaths, or until you feel the difference. Over time, through this simple self-healing technique, you can make good progress even with some of the symptoms described earlier.

Stress and trauma are often unavoidable in our modern world, but we can give our body the parasympathetic buffer zone it needs to handle things better. And we can do the work to clear away our backlog of past distress. The breath should become your best ally to accomplish this. In the safe environment of our seminars we do a more powerful, in-depth conscious breathing session under the guidance of trained breathwork facilitators. We lie down and breathe for about an hour with more-than-usual volume and intensity. Don't try this at home until you are well experienced with it, but you can safely do twenty-minute sessions on your own with good results.

The oxygenation of cells and the renewed energy flow achieved through in-depth breathwork trigger the body's self-cleansing and repair mechanisms in a very pleasant and powerful way. Even one session can produce results that are real and remarkable. In later sessions, we can more actively direct the breath to specific areas of need in the body and can combine breathwork with other holistic therapies. Good breathing is so central to every part of our lives. Enter into regular breathwork and you will transform your health and your life—guaranteed! ▨

Fight-or-flight only? Michael Grant White likes to add these additional catchphrases to the two famous words that describe the action of the Sympathetic Nervous System (SNS). His full list is: *Fight, Flight, Freeze, Fake it, Stumble, Mumble, or Fun!* Freezing is akin to "playing possum" or too scared to move.

Mike adds, "Fun is anything from snickering to guffaws, to high-adrenaline sports like skiing. It stimulates the SNS, but is naturally balanced with an adequate parasympathetic response (PNS). Anxiety drugs lessen the SNS, but they can diminish the fun aspects and tend to numb us out. To maintain healthy fun, we need to strengthen the PNS, and then the SNS naturally backs off without hindering its healthy aspects."

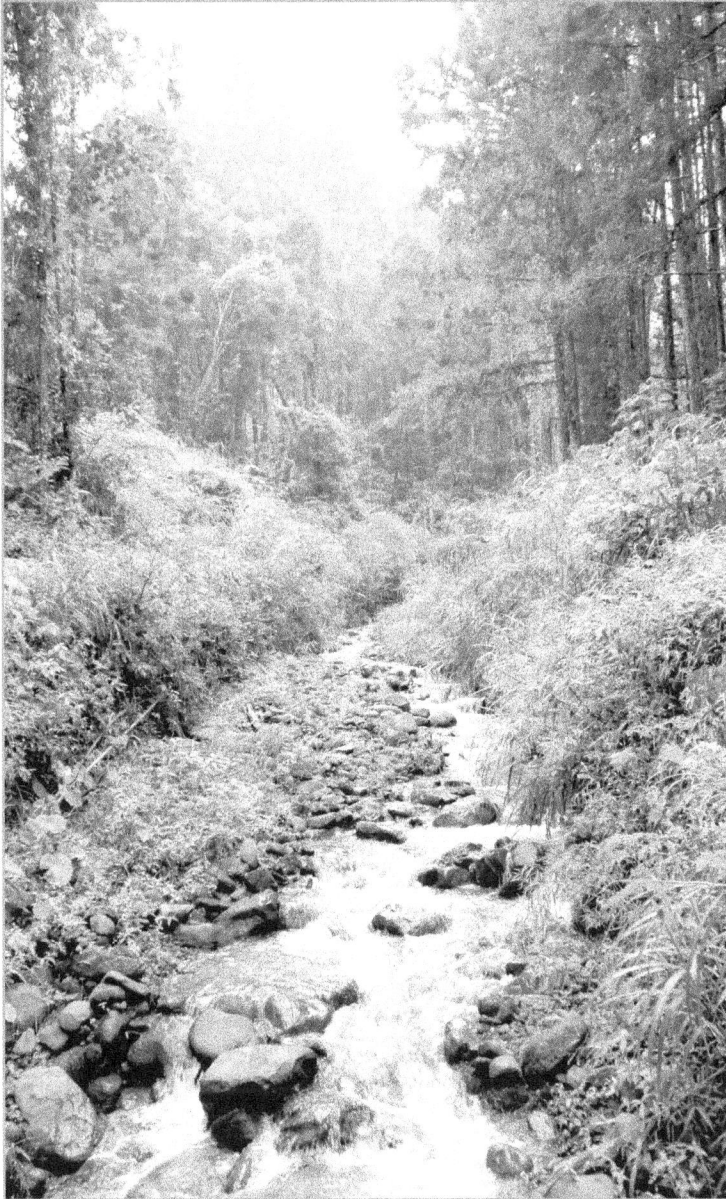

Oxygen Is Life!
It Does More Than You Think

Michael Grant White

Oxygen is life's first food. In proper balance, it vitalizes our body, calms the mind, and stabilizes the nervous system. Without oxygen we cannot absorb important vitamins, minerals, and nutrients. When our cells lack oxygen, they weaken and die. Without oxygen, nothing works very well at all!

Oxygen (O_2) and glucose sugars ($C_6H_{12}O_6$) create energy for use in the body through metabolism in the form of high-energy phosphate bonds, especially adenosine triphosphate (ATP), the primary energy currency of our cells. Water (H_2O) dissolves carbon dioxide (CO_2) and facilitates the hydrolysis (breakdown for use) of these energy-yielding phosphate bonds. Preliminary research demonstrates that ATP may be an analog to one aspect of what many call *qi* or *chi*, *prana*, *élan vital*, *pneuma*, or life-force energy.

The American Heart Association states that over 1.5 million people die every year from heart conditions and that 70% of our population has some evidence of heart problems. Most heart attacks originate from the heart's failure to receive adequate oxygen. Of course, maintaining one's arteries and capillaries for easy blood passage is important, but the fastest way to get oxygen right now is to breathe better.

Hypoxia (oxygen starvation) causes sympathetic nervous system overstimulation, inviting heart-rate increase, adrenal activation, and many other physiological changes as our bodies sound the alarm. Emotional and physical stress, anxiety, danger, or emergency create high oxygen loss. During episodes of stress and following physical exertion, the body uses up its oxygen stores to bring the nervous system back into a parasympathetic balance.

Too much fight or flight can invite eventual cardiac troubles. Stress that never lets up causes the heart to work harder to get the oxygen it needs. In an oxygen-starved environment, it may eventually

Τhe essential element in air that carries the vital charge of chi turns out to be neither oxygen, nor nitrogen, nor any other gaseous chemical, but rather the negative ion—a tiny, highly active molecular fragment that carries a negative electrical charge equivalent to that of one electron. By contrast, pollutants such as dust, smoke, and toxic chemicals are borne on the air in the form of large, sluggish, poly-molecular ions that carry a positive charge....

In clean country air, the average ratio of negative to positive ions is about three to one. In polluted city air, it drops drastically to about one negative ion against 500 positive ions! The vitality of negative ions in air is also destroyed by air-conditioning, central heating and closed spaces....

In nature, air is naturally ionized by the action of short-wave electro-magnetic radiation from the sun and by other cosmic rays, which bombard air molecules and impart vital energy to the fragments. The movement and evaporation of large bodies of water also ionize the air above them.

A third method of natural ioniza-tion is the unobstructed flow of wind over wide-open spaces. The most potent atmospheric chi is thus found at high altitudes, where solar and cosmic radiation are strongest, winds are constant, and water takes the form of rushing streams and open lakes.

The Tao of Health, Sex and Longevity:
A Modern Practical Guide
to the Ancient Way
by Daniel P. Reid

collapse from overwork. Many stressful states can be partial-ly or completely neutralized through proper breathing devel-opment and function.

Fresh fruits, vegetables, and rainwater contain oxygen. Green is the color of chlorophyll, or liquid oxygen, so green vegetables and especially high-chlorophyll plants like blue-green algae contain the most oxygen. Meat contains no oxy-gen and is "used protein." The body must employ a large amount of energy to break meat down into amino acids so it can recycle these building blocks and create usable protein, like building a car from used parts.

Cakes, candies, cookies, all empty carbs, and sugar con-tain no oxygen. Cooked and processed foods and stagnant water contain little or none. I call these "negative foods" as they use up more oxygen than they give off. Processed sug-ars, white flour, unhealthy fats, french fries, and pizza are major oxygen robbers. You can offset some of this loss by eating pounds of fresh fruits and vegetables daily. Not por-tions—pounds. Taking digestive enzymes and oxygen-rich nutritional supplements can also help.

Contrary to popular opinion, oxygen may, but may not, cause the body to relax. Oxygen can assist the blood toward achieving a balanced pH level, but this does not ensure relaxation. More important factors that determine our relax-ation response are how the body takes in the oxygen, whether it reaches the cells, and whether the autonomic nervous system is enervated sympathetically (through upper-chest breathing) or parasympathetically (through lower-diaphragmatic breathing) or by a combination of both.

Insufficient oxygen in our cells causes pain to be experi-enced more acutely than when oxygen supplies are ample. But breathing more does not ensure an increased oxygen supply. Breathing too quickly may cause a lessened oxygen supply to the cells and create an oxygen/carbon dioxide imbalance, sending more oxygen to the plasma but less to the cells. Carbon dioxide, due to its relationship with global warming, has received a lot of bad press, but we could not live without it. Carbon dioxide needs to be at a certain level in the plasma before the cells will take up oxygen.

Oxygen makes up almost 50% of the earth's surface by weight, 42% of all healthy vegetation, 85% of sea-water, 46% of igneous rock, and 47% of non-chemicalized, aerated dry soil. Overall oxygen levels on the planet at sea level are at about 20.8%. However, in basements, polluted cities, poorly ventilated offices, airplanes, etc., oxygen levels are much lower.

A common misconception is that a hundred years ago atmospheric oxygen was much higher than it is today. According to the Scripps Institute, there is no atmospheric oxygen shortage. Water tests from 10,000-year-old glaciers prove that the oxygen supply hasn't changed much at all. The rain forests are a significant supplier of oxygen (about 10%), but the oceans with their many forms of blue-green algae are the major suppliers of the earth's oxygen. Polluting the seas is asking for rampant sickness and accelerated aging for everyone, including fish, whales, and dolphins.

When slow, deep breathing and moderate body motion is activated, there is an increased demand for oxygen molecules, which are taken up from the blood. The potential for neutralizing free radicals as they bond with this available oxygen may be greatly accelerated when regular breathing, slightly deeper but still easy, is included in a person's regular daily health routine.

Your lungs will deteriorate 9%–25% per decade (Framingham study, www.breathing.com/articles/clinical-studies.htm) unless you do something to maintain them. Exercise is mandatory. Excessive stress in exercising can actually cause breathing blocks that invite inadequate levels of oxygen. The more we tighten up the primary and accessory breathing muscles, the more we cause the alveoli in our lungs (where oxygen goes into the bloodstream) to clog up with waste products. This will impede the body's ability to absorb oxygen, we will slowly suffocate, and our life spans will shorten.

As our cells grow older, they lose their ability to carry oxygen. As the liver ages, it robs increasing amounts of oxygen reserves for detoxification, often leaving the other body systems with an oxygen shortage. When needed, the cells send signals to send more oxygen. Our brains need it most, so when oxygen is in short supply in the body, our brains suffer the consequences.

For optimum health, learn to breathe better—fuller, easier, deeper, slower. Eat more nutritious and oxygen-rich foods with more live enzymes to make sure you digest what you eat. And exercise moderately without excessive straining, gasping, or breath-heaving. When you exercise, remember that physical stress creates very high oxygen loss. If stress and conditioning helped the organism to survive, then why wouldn't athletes live to be at least 120? Stress can condition muscles, but that is not the key to longevity. Maximum oxygen and energy intake with minimal expenditure plus breathing volume and flow rate (Framingham study) are the keys to longevity. Gentle natural breathing, breathing development techniques, regular cleansing of toxins, and replenishment of energy stores seem to be the best means to a longer and more joyful, energetic, and peaceful life.

When oxygen levels are increased, the red blood cells pick up the extra oxygen and provide it to our body tissues. Waste gases and toxins are removed more efficiently and cells begin to function normally. Anaerobic viruses, bacteria, and fungi, unable to live in an oxygen-enriched environment, are defeated. Oxygen builds resistance to infections like yeast (*candida albicans*) that thrive in an oxygen-deficient environment. Oxygen helps to neutralize acids in our body, such as lactic acid resulting from muscle overload. Our body's chemical reactions are fired up due to the increased oxygen levels. We burn fat more efficiently. We feel better, our body is healthier, and we think more clearly. Here are more benefits:

- *Removes free radicals*
- *Reduces tissue swelling*
- *Increases neuronal energy metabolism in the brain*
- *Can create sustained cognitive improvement*
- *Wakes up sleeping (idling) brain cells that are metabolizing enough to stay alive but are not actively "firing"*
- *Enhances the body's ability to fight bacterial and viral infections*
- *Deactivates toxins and poisons (e.g., side effects from some chemotherapy, spider bites, air pollution, etc.)*
- *Enhances wound healing (stimulates new capillaries)*
- *Creates an immediate aerobic state*
- *Acts as an anti-inflammatory*

www.Breathing.com

Exhale!

What comes first, the inhale or the exhale? A chicken-or-egg question. Naturally, when we think of inhaling we think of filling the lungs, and with exhaling we think of emptying the lungs. Life starts with our very first inbreath and ends with our last outbreath. But in between, no doubt, it's a circle. Just for fun, let's look at the exhale in some other ways. Maybe we'll conclude that the exhale often comes first!

Think of the Big Bang as God's original out-breath when creating the cosmos. Now think of Genesis 2:7, *And the LORD God formed man of the dust of the ground, and breathed into his nostrils the Breath of Life; and man became a living soul.* With these two primal exhales, we think of expanding and giving life, rather than emptying.

Now think of blowing through a pipe. Because there are holes at both ends, we empty it while filling it. It's a process of giving while receiving.

Here's another point of view. What do you say when you see a glorious sunset? *"Aaahhhhhhh!"* Now you see the exhale as relaxation, contemplation of beauty, a way of opening up and bringing some of that beauty into yourself and merging with it.

Here are some other exhaling sounds that we could say are counterproductive. A forced *Whhoooo!"* through pursed lips. An exasperated *"Huhhhh!"* (or its nasal variety) when you're mad. A *"Humphffffff!"* when you've been insulted and you're stomping out the door. What about a gasp? This is sucking in and holding the breath out of fear, danger, or pain. Let's examine these a little closer.

As a breathworker and bodyworker, I've learned a lot over the years from studying breathing physiology and using the breath as a therapeutic tool. I've come to respect the exhale as something more than what meets the eye.

The exhale releases carbon dioxide from the lungs. But did you know that most of the body's toxins are, or should be, mixed with methane gas in the liver and expelled though the exhale? Did you know that fatigue and other ill-health conditions often result from a build-up of toxins not released sufficiently through the exhale? How does the body handle an overload of toxins? One common way is by wrapping and buffering the toxins in fat cells and storing them until the body can deal with them properly. *"Ho ho ho!"* as jolly round Santa would say, which reminds us that laughing, *"Ha ha ha!"* is a very healthful exhale indeed!

Have you ever seen the red faces of people when they're lifting heavy weights? They're probably doing a "Whoooooo" through tight, pursed lips, or a *"SSSsss!"* or *"FFFfff!"* through teeth or lips, or worse, they're holding their breath during the exertion with eyes popping and heart pounding. Can any of that be good for the system?

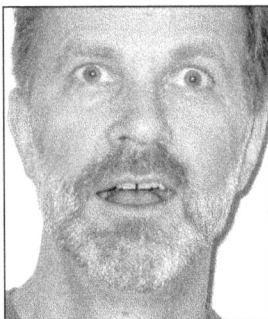

The *Aaahhhhh!* Relaxed, gazing-at-sunset exhale.

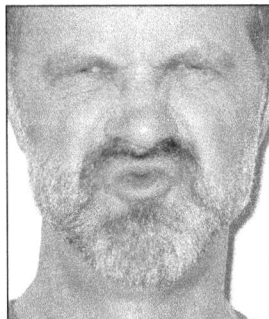

The *Whoooooo!* Tight-lipped, forced exhale. Bad for your body!

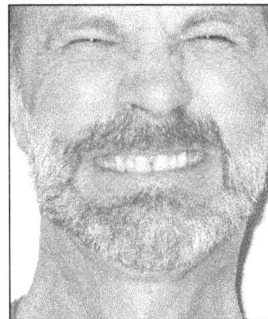

The *Ssssssssss!* Exhaling through teeth. See its cousin, next page.

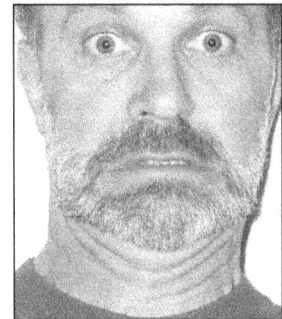

The Gasp. Not an exhale. Often used when exhaling would be better.

During a breathwork session, we do a cleansing breath, which includes an open-mouthed, relaxed-jaw *"Haaaaaaa!"* Picture a wave crashing on the shore, freely spilling its momentum. In your body, the wave is the ideal inhale, filling the lower torso first. Next the wave rolls up, spreading your ribs and rippling up your spine. Without pausing at the top, you exhale, neither pushing out nor holding back. All your muscles relax and tensions go. Gravity takes over.

Let's revisit the jaw thing. With those angry, insulted exhales, you can imagine they are accompanied by a clenched jaw. Fight-or-flight, stress, and withheld anger can increase jaw tension, sometimes chronically so. Right now, place your fingertips on your cheekbones, then go down about half an inch into the meaty muscle just below. Press in. It hurts, doesn't it? That's your jaw-flapping muscle, and it's tight on most people. Massage it with slow circular movements. Allow your jaw to hang down more and more.

Now imagine a totally jaw-dropping experience. Let's say you're Nicholas Cage in *National Treasure*, and you just saw the billions of dollars of loot. You might breathe in with surprise, but your next exhale would be totally relaxed and your jaw would be hanging as the reality of it all sank in.

Now lie down and do the things just described, especially that letting-go exhale through the mouth. Roll the inhale up from the belly, then let it all spill out. Hear the wave crashing on the shore. Feel your muscles, organs, skeletal system, and nervous system all relaxing. This is an effective detoxing and cleansing breath.

Pursing the lips will make you hold back and re-internalize some of those toxins and some of the carbon dioxide. A thick, fat tongue or a tight jaw can do the same. Others have a very reserved and almost timid exhale, *"hhhhhhhhhh!"* or *"fffffffffff!"* These can calm the system, but they won't necessarily detox it. Don't push out on the exhale, which can make you dizzy and create an oxygen/carbon dioxide imbalance. Just let go.

After about ten of these, you may feel aches and pains coming to your awareness that you didn't realize you had. Stored tension goes numb after a while, when your nervous system realizes you're not paying attention. So this is a good chance to reacquaint yourself with your body and do some self-healing. My friend KRS Edstrom, an alternative health practitioner, has a program on CD called *Defeat Pain*. [See www.askkrs.com.] In it, she asks you to visualize the painful area dissipating and spreading out in concentric rings like when a pebble hits the water. "You feel the pain, you allow the waves to spread." Try this along with your smooth exhales. You'll be communicating with your tension. It will understand and let go.

I use a similar technique when giving a massage. If I'm going to press on someone's tense, painful muscle, I'll do it only while they're expressing one of these relaxing exhales. Your first instinct when someone is pressing on a sore spot would be to gasp, hold your breath, and tighten up even more. Doing the opposite, exhaling with an open-mouthed *"Haaaaaaaaaa..."* while relaxing the muscle, is

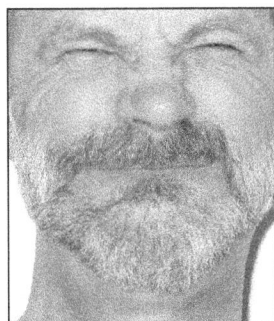

The *FFFfff!* Why put your body through this kind of an exhale?

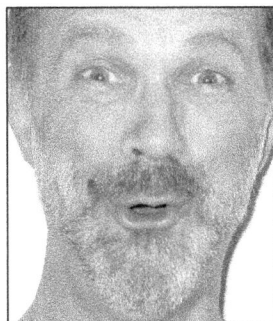

A thin person's *Ho ho ho!* Next to air, jolliness is the #1 health tonic.

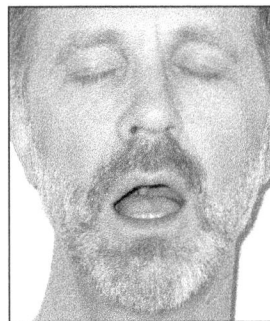

This looks like snoring, but it's the ideal *Haaaaaaa* exhale for breathwork.

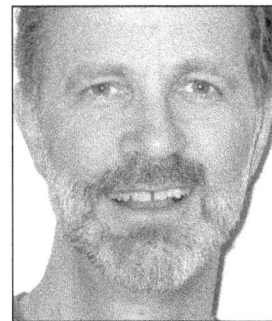

OK—rubber face back to normal. What a way to make a living!

very effective. I don't use the nasal equivalent of this until toward the end of the massage, because I want to encourage a more voluminous, cleansing, detoxing exhale.

Earlier, we visualized a pipe with the exhale coming in at one end and exiting at the other. Now imagine that the pipe is the nozzle of a blacksmith's bellows. The inhale is like the filling of the bellows. With the exhale, you can direct the flow of air and energy to a specific area of the body for healing.

Those who practice hands-on healing techniques and other energy work are familiar with sending energy through their hands in conjunction with their exhale. You can add further visualizations to this. For instance, as you breathe in, open your crown and let the universal energy flow into you. Now charge it with the love of your heart, then send it down your arms and out your hands. Energy follows thought. Love charges and attracts more energy.

For self-healing, direct the flow of energy to your own areas of chronic pain, emotional turmoil, poor circulation, etc. Feed yourself energy, especially where you need it most. Add love and letting-go to the mixture. It works.

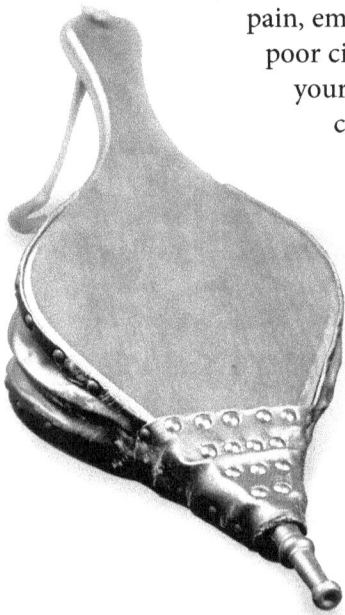

Recent studies in mainland China show that when deep breathing is performed with the mind firmly focused on a certain part of the body, that part registers a strong electric charge and grows warm. This accords well with the findings of Dr. Chang Rui, director of the imperial medical institute during the Southern Sung Dynasty (1127–1279):

> *Mind is the leader of energy. Where mind goes, energy follows. When a certain part of the body is ailing, use the mind to draw energy to the affected area and it will correct the condition.*

> *The Tao of Health, Sex and Longevity: A Modern Practical Guide to the Ancient Way* by Daniel P. Reid

In our breathwork seminars, we go even deeper into a letting-go series of exhales, along with well-tuned inhales, of course. The breathing process we use takes people into deeper levels of releasing old injuries and traumas, even emotional stress and hurt, even negative thoughts and attitudes.

Our brain and internal nervous system and our cells themselves hold the memory of past trauma, which can show up as tension, fight-or-flight responses, protectiveness in parts of the body, or emotional and mental withdrawal. It's as if the burdensome events of the past get backlogged just like those toxins, sometimes to a dangerous point of overload.

Let breathing, in conjunction with other natural healing methods, free you from the burdens of your past. Oxygen intake, combined with glorious detoxing exhales, will provide you with more energy for your pursuit of happiness!

Sound & Light:
Energy Follows Thought

In the last chapter, we mentioned the Big Bang and the creation of man in Genesis. Let's look at the first day of Creation. In Genesis 1:3 we read, "And God said: 'Let there be light.' And there was light." In Latin this is "Lux fiat!" From these immortal first words, the noun *fiat* has come to mean "a command or act of will that creates something without, or as if without, further effort. An authoritative determination." God used the sound of His voice coupled with a powerful intent to create light, and from light He went on to create all the other manifestations of His design. John's Gospel begins with, "In the beginning was the Word." The Greek term for *word*, *Logos*, is defined as "reason...the controlling principle of the universe." The essence and potential (light and energy) came into manifestation through the spoken word (sound and intent).

Other examples in the New Testament demonstrate Jesus' mastery of these principles. With "Peace be still!" (Mark 4:36) he rebuked the waters and calmed the stormy sea. When his good friend Lazarus died, Jesus prayed to his Father (he established the connection and marshaled his forces) and cried out in a loud voice, "Lazarus, come forth!" (John 11:37-40), resurrecting Lazarus from the dead.

Energy follows thought, especially when the thought is spoken with authoritative determination. Then why doesn't it work when a mom is trying to get her teenager out of bed with, "Joey, come forth!" The determination on the mom's part is there, and probably the loud voice as well. Perhaps some of the authority has worn off, but then again, there was Jesus' great mastery in marshaling light through sound to manifest his will. The potential for developing this mastery is there for all of us. It's part of what this book is all about.

Later, in Part Two, Chapter 13, we'll learn how to conduct a marvelous ancient healing ritual that combines breath, light, sound, and water, called an *Essene Rebirth*. Seven people hold one floating in warm water, with one holding the head and three pairs of two holding the body. Sunlight or colored artificial light may be used to charge the water beforehand. Herbs and/or aromatherapy may be employed. Sacred syllables are intoned by the seven on behalf of the one receiving the healing.

Spiritual light is invoked through the words and focused intention of the seven. The participant receives the harmonized impetus from these natural forces—breath, light, sound, and water—magnified and amplified, not through machines, but through the physical, mental, emotional, and spiritual intent and energy passing through the seven. Several times I have been on the receiving or giving ends of this ritual, and it is truly an indescribable, transcendent experience.

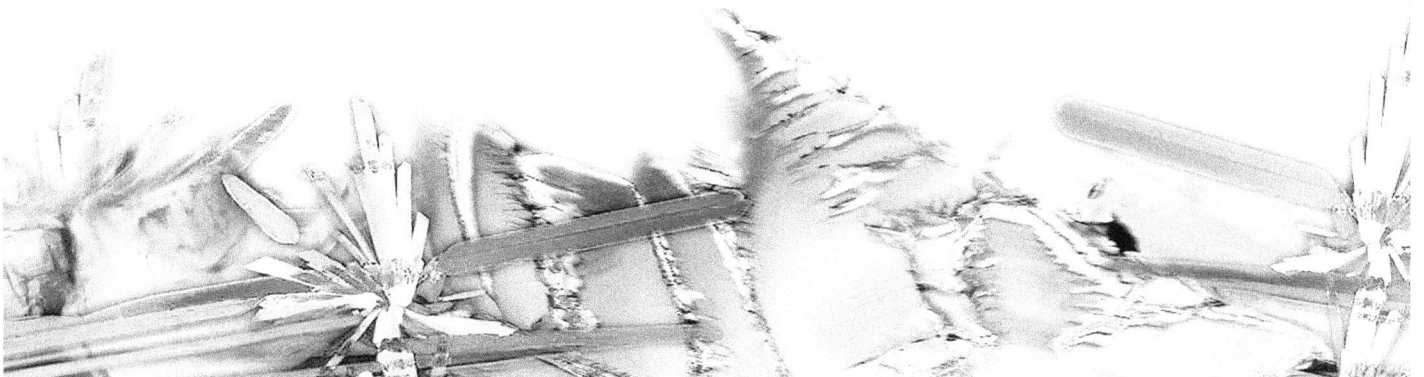

Prior to teaching us this ritual, Katherine the Healer guides us to use invocations to clear the room and create a sacred space. She says, "Remember always during the process that all is thought. All that is necessary for thought to be realized in physical manifestation is verbalization. The word is what *is*, thus the verbal clearing of the room or the water before the rebirth."

The power of intention to create change and facilitate healing is the subject of many books and a key tool taught by self-improvement speakers. In Part Three, Chapter 2, you can read from Sol Luckman's groundbreaking work, *Conscious Healing*, for a glimpse at the science now coming to the fore as to how our DNA are receptors for, and operate through the agency of, sound and light. Within this chapter, read also the excerpts from Steve Guettermann and Gia Combs-Ramirez for introductions on the use of clear intent and energy medicine.

Prior to doing breathwork at our seminars, we verbalize our goals for the session with a partner and scan our physical bodies, mental and emotional states, and memories for issues and areas we would like to target for healing. [See *Goal Setting* in Appendix.] This is a good tool for setting intentions. When people are new to self-healing work and to breathwork—and we often see this in our lives in general—we tend to take a more passive approach. Our experiences can be dramatic and we often find it enough of a challenge just to hold on for the ride and get through it. As we build confidence through practice, we begin to learn how to direct the process more and how to combine our words and our wills to take a more active role with our healing endeavors.

In explaining the nebulous concept of intentionality to people, I often refer to Bettie Eadie's experience described in her book *Embraced by the Light*, called the most profound and complete description of a near-death experience ever recorded. Her first concern after leaving her body on the hospital bed was for her children. She registered the thought "I must see my children" with a high level of emotional intensity, and instantly her spirit-body was transported to her home, where she could observe her family. As Edie's experience demonstrates, any thought is made more powerful when there is a strong feeling behind it, and this form of navigation is not reserved for after death. We can use verbalization and intent (will power) to accomplish it. Words from my dad come to mind: "You've got to apply yourself!"

Edgar Cayce said that sound would become the medicine of the future. Further advances in the understanding of our energetic, electromagnetic, sound-and-light bodies are forthcoming daily. And yet, the ancient and indigenous people understood and were naturally drawn to working with these forces. We can harmonize the old with the new, the mystical with the scientific. And we can holistically embrace the continuum of who we are, from physical to mental to emotional to spiritual. The processes and therapies presented here do just that.

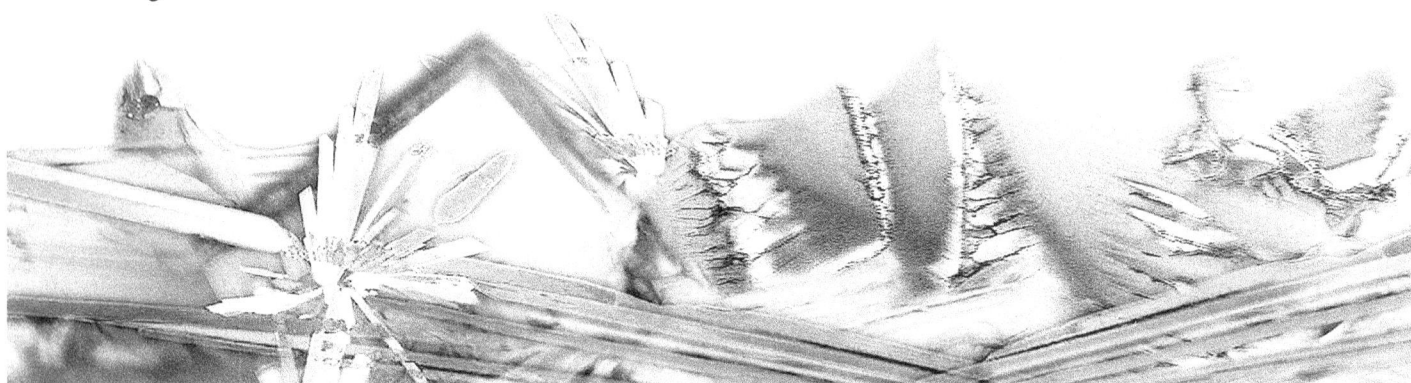

Our Crystalline Nature

Steve Guettermann

Western science and medicine now realize that the human body is, among other things, a crystalline operating system. As studies continue, it is becoming clearer that our crystal-colloidal matrix is the biological structure that allows for the most rapid communication between the mind, brain, and body, predominantly through electrical impulses.

A laser beam cuts through steel, yet uses less energy than the average light bulb. What makes the laser's power so palpable? Concentrated energy to a single purpose. As human beings, we can choose to use our energy to either light up a room or cut through steel. However, we cannot do one or the other, or anything else with real impact, if we send mixed signals to ourselves and to everything around us.

One of the strongest sources of mixed signals is our own internal dialogue—our thoughts. As the silently spoken word, what we say to ourselves radiates from our inner world to the outside. It contributes to our expressed intent—for good or ill. Our crystalline system works as a semi-conductor—a certain amount of energetic push, or amplitude, is necessary to move a signal along the system. If our thoughts and intentions are not clear, they are not high-powered. If our thoughts or actions don't excite us, we never generate the power (the feeling) necessary to activate the energy around us into a creative partner in our intent. Our system clogs up and we get a lot of error messages, "That does not compute!"

Taking command of our internal dialogue can play a key role in focusing energy, amplifying intent, and creating the excitement necessary to direct our crystalline structure to radiate power into the undifferentiated (ready-to-go) energy around us. How we talk to ourselves about ourselves and about everything and everyone around us can create a communication quagmire or a springboard to excitement, awareness, and fulfillment. It is our choice to qualify and quantify that dialogue. We have total control over it!

Top performers in every discipline know this well. Confidence and charisma radiate from them. They spin setback into motivation. Most of today's leaders, inventors, and trend-setters are people who let their internal and external dialogues translate into focused action. They program their crystalline structure for self-fulfillment through focused intent.

For a quick boost, try a high-powered, focused internal dialogue session (an internal pep talk) that is consistent with your heart's intent, and carry yourself in a way that projects fulfillment into the energy around you. Coupled with exercise and meditation, this process will clean your crystalline structure so intended thought can flow through you with power and result in fulfillment. ▨

Steve Guettermann trains people in peak performance, yoga, and meditation. A freelance writer, he worked closely with Jack Schwarz, author of the pioneering work *Human Energy Systems*. E-mail migratoryanimal@earthlink.net. Reprint from *Natural Life News & Directory*, Sept–Oct 2005.

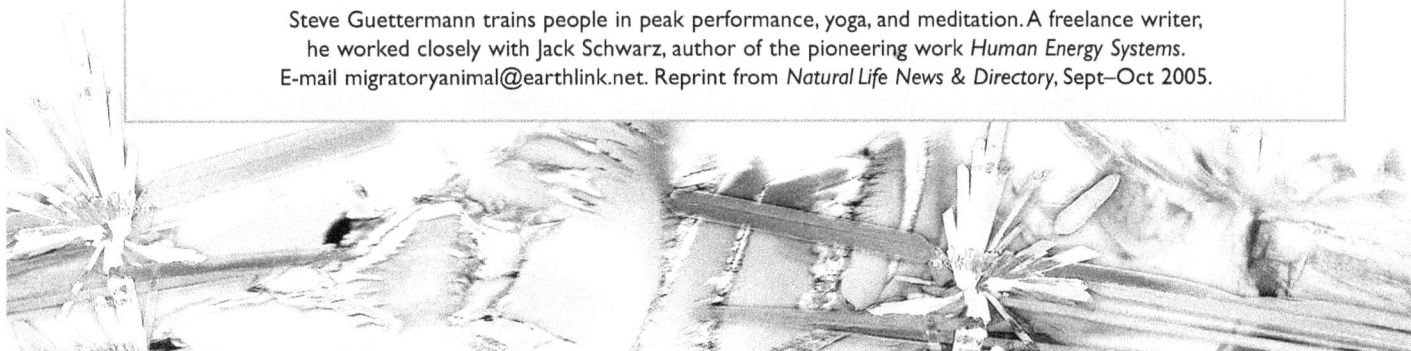

Crystalline Consciousness Technique™

The Science of Energy Healing ~ *Gia Combs-Ramirez*

Crystalline Consciousness Technique (CCT) is a new modality in the field of energy medicine that heals the energy body and works with the power of intention. In his book, *The Power of Intention*, author Wayne Dyer quotes Carlos Castaneda as saying, "Intent is a force that exists in the universe." In CCT, conscious intention works with that universal force, acting to influence, alter, shape, modify, and create the energy patterns that organize and shape reality in a positive way. CCT practitioners use it on themselves, clients, and for healing in group dynamics. One of the unexpected results of CCT is the creation of stable energy fields that provide greater protection for people who are ultrasensitive to crowds, fluorescent lights, or other electromagnetic interference. Practitioners have reported a greater sense of connection and ease in relationships. Those in the healing arts have found that CCT enhances their modalities.

In our daily lives of sensory overwhelm, we rarely get to observe the power of intention as it shapes and directs our lives. When it is spoken to a body that is quiet, open, receptive, and unified, it is often deeply felt as the vibration of the words penetrate tissue. Intention provides the organizing dynamic for the cells of the body. We often know what we *don't* want in our lives, but our bodies need a positive direction and sense of forward movement for growth and health. Intention answers the question, "What *do* I want?"

TIPS FOR WORKING WITH INTENTION

When you state an intention, the universe responds. How the intention becomes manifested is part of the great mystery of living. Below are some tips for becoming more efficient at working with intention.

1. Be conscious about your intentions. Allow yourself time in the morning to get calm and quiet. Focus your mind on your heart, then ask yourself, "What would I like to see happen today?"

2. Always state your intention in the positive. Many of us are used to focusing only on what we don't want.

3. Be explicit. Many of us use shortcuts in our communication, implying certain things without actually saying them.

4. Keep a journal. Observe and write down what begins to shift and change in your life. As you do, you'll understand yourself better, leading to clearer intentions. At the same time, you'll begin to trust the universe to respond to your intentions.

5. Bring your awareness to others. Intentions empower! Invite your children or your spouse to state their intentions before starting a new endeavor. When talking to people who tend to complain, invite them to shift their focus by asking, "What would you have liked to see happen?"

Gia Combs-Ramirez is cofounder of Crystalline Consciousness Technique and teaches classes in the science of energy healing. E-mail Gia at rramblerg@mac.com. Reprint from *Natural Life News & Directory*, Sept–Oct 2005.

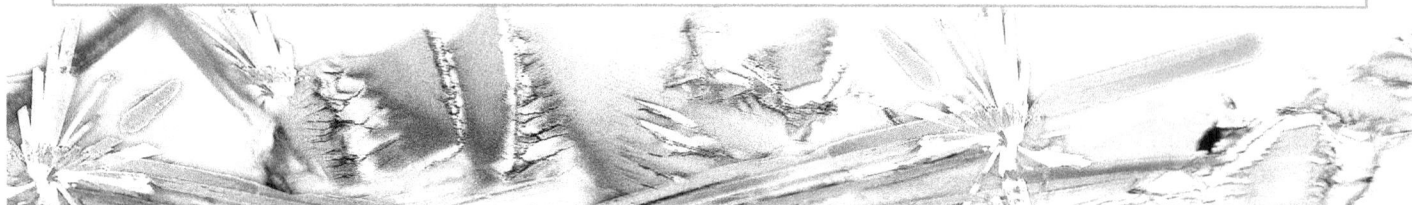

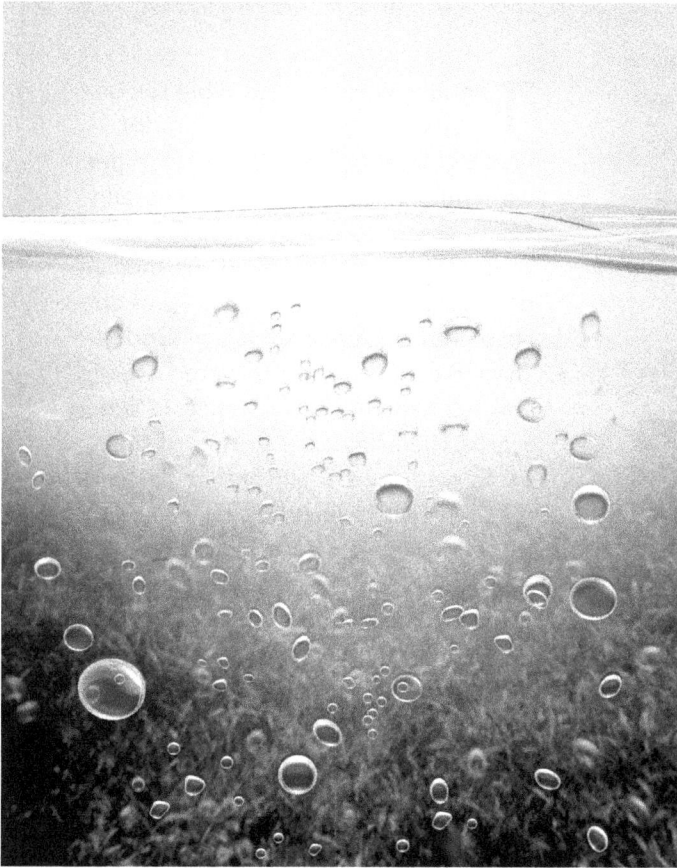

Water & Earth
Our Body

"The earth was a formless void and darkness covered the face of the deep, while a wind from God swept over the face of the waters."
(Genesis 1:2)

Air, spirit, light, sound, energy, and electricity all need to ride on something to be perceived. By themselves, they are almost unmanifest. They need a medium, they need to animate a body made of water and earth, the cups that hold and deliver these subtler forces. Pure and beautiful by nature, water and earth passively absorb the burdens of man's miscreations, attempting to purify them, until their own burdens become too great. We see this on the planet and within our bodies and cells.

Earth and water want to cleanse us and make us whole again. They continually refresh and renew us. In its desire to heal us, nature also provides, through the marriage of earth and water, a cornucopia of herbs, plants, and their essences. What do they desire from us in return? They want us to magnify, amplify, and glorify their work, respond to their giving nature in kind, and flood them in return with the subtler animating forces of air, spirit, light, sound, and energy. This is the cosmic dance and interplay of the elements. Cups filling and spilling, giving and receiving, as each one says to the other, "Drink me while I am drinking thee."

Breathing, praying and praising, chanting and intoning, drumming, sharing love and gratitude, laughing and having fun, enjoying nature, entering into rituals of purification—all the ways we cycle spirit back into matter—are registered by and ring clearly and gratefully on the water and the earth. They too are thirsty. It is our role and duty as spiritual beings to infuse our planet and our bodies with a constant flow of these subtler forces. They are the conductors; we provide the juice. Yet our bodies are 70% water and the earth is 70% water, so we are not only the cup and the drink, but also the singing energy and the vibration, the consciousness that infuses them.

Now was all that clear as mud—water and earth mixed?

Dr. Masaru Emoto's work on the impressionability of water is now world famous. Emoto has shown that water is an excellent medium for healing, for holding a charge of sunlight, sacred sounds and music, and good vibrations. The *Essene Rebirth* described in Part II combines all of these mediums with water for healing. We know about the body's need for water and we're beginning to value the difference between bad, good and great water. [See *Hexagonal Water* in Resources for a summary of Dr. Emoto's work and Dr. Mu Shik Jhon's work on the structure of water.] We can now partner with the waters we all swim in (from our cells to the planet) and help this element fulfill its reason for being, which is to heal, to nurture, and to give life. Take every opportunity to drink in its blessings and to bless it in return.

The earth element is also a great super-conductor of energy and electricity. For good or ill, it absorbs and responds to sound, light, words, feelings, and intent. This is more easily illustrated in its negative aspect. People can literally be made sick from negative energy that is directed powerfully at them.

The minerals and chemicals in the body serve as electrical generators and conductors for the repair of our DNA. The earth's electromagnetic forces sustain our life; they can heal us when magnified and amplified. Electric fields are everywhere—the earth and our bodies swim in them. For a primer on these subjects, see *The Earth's and Our Body's Health-Enhancing Electric Fields* by John C. Ledbetter (Part Three, Chapter 2). John explains how the flow of these electrical forces is responsible for the success of many of today's Complementary Alternative Medicine (CAM) approaches, such as acupuncture, breathwork, bodywork, and energy work.

Healing yourself will also heal the waters and the earth. Call it the ripple effect. The waters and the earth will also heal you. So make liberal use of water through hydrotherapy, pure water hydration, doing breathwork in water, charging your drinking and bathing water with worded invocations, sound, sunlight and herbs, swimming in pure lakes and oceans, and in many other ways.

You can access the power of the earth by visiting sacred sites and healing spas, hiking in the mountains, doing your choice of natural therapies, or practicing the oriental *chi* disciplines. Freely partake of earth's abundance by eating whole live foods, drinking liquid chlorophyll, and enjoying aromatherapy essences.

All of these can amplify, carry, and deliver to you, and to those you love and serve, the subtle powers that flow through water and earth for healing.

The first words of the Bible tell us that water was the medium for God's creation of the world: "Darkness was over the surface of the deep, and God's breath swept over the water." Water was the energy and the medium of sharing. The act of creation was an absolutely pure expression of God's sharing essence, and the water itself was imbued with this essence. In other words, the primordial waters of the earth were free of any and all destructive or negative energies. There could be no drowning. There could be no floods or tidal waves. Water could only heal, nurture, and help.

www.KabbalahWater.com

Chi moves around with the wind and sits still in water (Feng Shui literally means "wind and water"), and it shows its various faces in the five elements—fire, earth, water, metal, and wood. Thanks to this Chi, all aspects of our environment are connected and have a direct impact on our mind, body, spirit... and even our love life. When Chi is fresh flowing, it nourishes us, but when it's blocked or stagnant, it can have bad effects on many areas of our lives, including relationships, career, creativity, health and money matters.

Let the Love Flow, Feng Shui Style, from JDate.com

Clear, Clean Water!

Water is second only to air as the key element in our life. Our very existence depends upon the adequacy and proper balance of the water within us. This refers to both the amount of water we consume and our ability to absorb it. The proper water balance depends upon the interaction of water with sodium and protein in our bodies. Salt and protein move water to where it should be and help to keep it there.

About 70% of our total body weight is water. Did you know that the lungs are 90% water, the brain is 76% water, and even our bones are 25% water. With 75% of all muscles and 91.5 of blood plasma being made up of water, water's importance becomes even more obvious. Water replenishment typically comes from three sources: 60% from fluid replacement, 30% from food, and 10% from metabolism. A 9%–12% drop in body weight as a result of water loss can be fatal. Within our cells lies 67% percent of the water in our bodies, yet this is in constant flux with our extracellular fluids. Our bodies constantly compensate for the fluctuating moisture content in our environment. Perspiration (especially during exercise) and excessive loss of water through diet must also be factored in.

In *Your Body Knows Best,* Ann Louise Gittleman recommends the consumption of eight glasses of water per day, between meals. Although our primary source of water is drinking water, we also receive water from the air we breathe and through our skin. The air's moisture level is crucial to the health of sinus tissue, bronchial tubes, and lungs. Drinking additional water during the relatively dry days of winter and the hot days of summer helps to maintain water balance. While there is typically more precipitation in winter than in summer, less water is available in winter air because of colder temperatures.

The body's loss of water through urination is increased by drinking caffeine or alcohol. These diuretics stimulate the kidneys to excrete more urine, depleting us not only of water but also of vital water-soluble vitamins (C and B complex) and important minerals (calcium, magnesium, potassium, sodium, chloride, and zinc). For every cup of coffee or glass of alcohol you consume, replenish the water lost by drinking an additional glass of water.

The water we drink has come under increasing scrutiny in recent years. Chlorination of municipal water supplies has been common since 1908. This method of water disinfection is effective in neutralizing bacteria and other water-borne pathogens, but some bacteria are necessary for the healthy functioning of our digestive system. Pure spring water is the obvious solution to our water concerns; however, maintaining our water in a pristine state is not easy. Water contaminants such as pesticides, fertilizers, industrial pollution, and naturally occurring compounds can compromise the purity of spring water. The challenge of how to clean water has been addressed in many ways. Carbon filters, ultraviolet light, and reverse osmosis are but a few. Water and life are so synonymous that we must be cognizant of anything that alters our water.

In one form or another, water is constantly entering, flowing through, and exiting our bodies. Our blood, bile, perspiration, tears, and lymphatic fluids are all dependent upon abundant water in proper balance. Water delivers nutrients to our cells and carries away unwanted wastes. Colon hydrotherapy, the irrigation and cleansing of the colon, is effective for detoxifying and hydrating the tissues, and it can aid in the absorption of water throughout the body. The cleansed tissue can more readily absorb both water and nutrients from our food.

Clear, clean water is essential to the proper functioning of every cell in our bodies, our digestion and elimination systems, and our overall health. So pay attention to your fluid intake and let the water flow as you cleanse yourself both within and without.

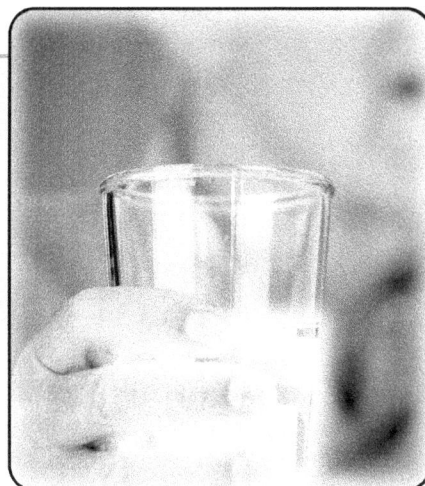

Georgia Cold, Healing Waters Colon Hydrotherapy, Bozeman, Montana
Reprint from *Natural Life News & Directory,* Jan–Feb 2003

"Getting the War Out"

NEW PARADIGMS FOR HEALING POST-TRAUMATIC STRESS

Denis W. Ouellette

Not many of us get through life without bumps, grinds and dents along the way. They say that stress becomes trauma when the injury takes up residence—when an event was so overwhelming for us that we can't seem to recover from it. We think of soldiers coming back from war, but some of that war never seems to leave them.

As a bodyworker and breath-worker, I've worked with releasing stress and tension from bodies for 30 years. I've learned to trust the body's ability to self-heal, and that many problems that seem mental and emotional, are locked and blocked in the body's cells and nervous system too. They say that 75% of the time, doctor's can't find anything wrong when patients come to them with complaints. They call this psychosomatic, i.e., "it's all in your mind." Yet stress and the effects of trauma are often the cause, and mind-oriented talk therapies, and/or psychoactive drugs, have produced less-than-complete results in many cases. Let's examine emerging natural therapies, and new paradigms for understanding the key role that somatic experience (trusting the body's innate self-healing powers) plays in resolving the effects of trauma.

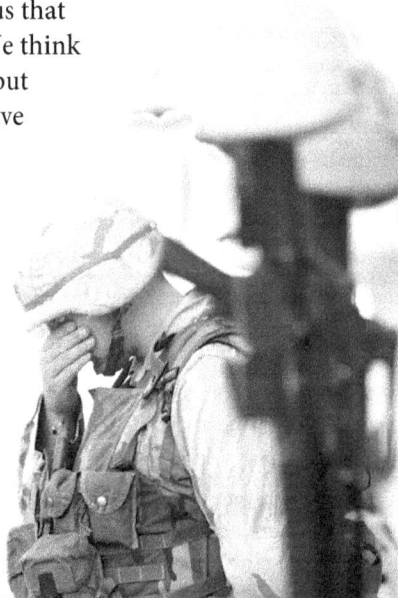

I was giving a lady from the east coast a massage recently and we got to talking about her son, who recently returned from Iraq. "I wish you could work on my son," she said, "that Walter Reed Hospital patched up his

---

RAPID EYE TECHNOLOGY (RET)

My oldest son is a Marine and I am a proud Marine mom. At 21, he was sent over to Iraq for his first tour there. He was away for 7 months. When he came back to the states and was able to spend his 30 days of leave at home, I became very aware that all was not well. When darkness fell, he was absolutely haunted, and for 30 days straight, he would have to leave and go out with his friends to drink. Many nights he would not come home.

It was very sad to watch. He was a profound alcoholic and in such a state of remorse. I finally asked him about what happened over there. He began to sob and said bluntly, "I don't remember, it's as if I was never there. I remember leaving and I remember coming back." How do you help a matter of the heart like this?

Some time after this, I was referred to RET with the hope this would help my son. I found a technician in his area and signed him up. I asked my son to just do this for me on faith, as neither of us had ever heard of it. After only five sessions, a profound change had occurred, evident as he began to spend weekends fishing or with family and friends. He was able to sleep at night.

His second tour to Iraq came quickly and I was very glad to see such healing had occurred before he left. I honestly believe the RET saved my son's life, for if he had gone to Iraq on that second tour in the same shape he was when he came home from the first, I am not sure he would have lived through it. During his second tour to Iraq, he called aunts, uncles and grandmas, very much more connected than before. I am grateful every day for the RET and what it did for my son and our family.

— Jacque Chapman

wounds but didn't do a thing for his psyche... Boy, does HE need anger management!"

I also worked on a psychiatrist from a major-city veteran's hospital and I asked him what they do there for PTSD (Post-Traumatic Stress Disorder). He admitted that their approach was not enough, mostly using drugs and group therapy. He talked about how when there is shock or trauma, the neuropeptides (transmitters in the brain and nervous system) get frozen. Locked "at the scene of the crime," so to speak, replaying the event, or "stuck in emergency mode," which is the body's fight-or-flight response, and unable to unwind and re-balance, resulting in the many, complex symptoms of PTSD: flashbacks, hypervigilance, dissociation, memory loss, and a disconnect from parts of the body, avoidance of restimulating experiences. (See the sidebar for a longer list of symptoms.) If not resolved, coping with trauma can evolve into bouts with depression, anxiety and addictions. This doctor talked about how the Alpha or Beta blockers commonly used for PTSD can blunt the memory and block the release of excess hormones (adrenaline, cortisol); but still, he said, "you've got to get the feelings out."

We talked about how the frontal cortex of the brain doesn't fully develop until the age of 28. That's the rational brain, responsible for long-range planning, global thinking, and "fuzzy logic," which is the ability to consider a host of variables, and how sad it is that soldiers (and other young trauma victims) may have this brain-maturation process interrupted. It reminded me of the statistic that 40% of the homeless in this country are Vietnam vets, with brains only capable of living in "survival mode." Back in the 70s, there was no PTSD diagnosis and little understanding or resources for soldiers returning from an unpopular war.

Let's look at how Dr. Peter Levine, a

TYPICAL PTSD SYMPTOMS

❑ Abrupt mood swings, e.g., rage reactions or temper tantrums, shame
❑ Addictive behaviors (overeating, drinking, drugs, etc.)
❑ Amnesia or forgetfulness
❑ Attention difficulties: ADD, ADHD, etc.
❑ Attraction to dangerous situations
❑ Avoidance behavior (avoiding certain circumstances and phobias)
❑ Chronic fatigue or very low physical energy
❑ Constriction (tightness in body parts)
❑ Compulsion to re-enact actions or circumstances that mirror the trauma
❑ Depression, feelings of impending doom
❑ Difficulty sleeping
❑ Diminished interest in life
❑ Dissociation (including denial)
❑ Exaggerated emotional and startle responses
❑ Exaggerated or diminished sexual activity
❑ Extreme sensitivity to light and sound
❑ Fear of dying, going crazy, or having a shortened life
❑ Feelings and behaviors of helplessness
❑ Feelings of detachment, alienation, and isolation, "living dead" feelings
❑ Fibromyalgia or skin disorders
❑ Frequent crying
❑ Hyper-vigilance (being "on guard" at all times)
❑ Hyperactivity or hyper-arousal
❑ Immune system problems or certain endocrine problems, i.e., thyroid malfunction or environmental sensitivities
❑ Inability to love, nurture, or bond with other individuals
❑ Inability to make commitments
❑ Intrusive imagery or flashbacks
❑ Loss of sustaining beliefs (spiritual, religious or interpersonal)
❑ Mental "blankness" or "spaciness"
❑ Nightmares or night terrors
❑ Panic attacks, anxiety or phobias
❑ Psychosomatic illnesses, particularly headaches, neck and back problems, asthma, digestive, spastic colon, or severe premenstrual syndrome
❑ Reduced ability to formulate plans or goals, living "hand-to-mouth"

Compiled from www.Breathing.com[2]
Copyright © Michael Grant White. All rights reserved.
and *Healing Trauma,* by Peter A. Levine, Ph.D.
See Recommended Reading.

psychologist and world leader in the somatic approach to trauma healing, describes the brain. We humans have three functioning parts of the brain, two of which we share with the animal kingdom. The survival brain, located in the lower rear, is sometimes called the reptilian brain and is our instinctual brain. From this part of the brain, life is viewed as either black or white, yes or no, friend or foe. Life is also only about needs in the present, i.e., "hand-to-mouth." This brain takes over in times of extreme stress.

With all mammals we share the mammalian brain, located in the center, which drives emotional bonding with others, caring for our young, etc. Only humans have the frontal cortex, the higher reasoning brain. Our three brains work together as an integrated whole when there is homeostasis, i.e., a fluid balance of communication and coordination. Dr. Levine describes how, when trauma occurs, the survival brain takes over and then, because of the overwhelm, is unable to reconnect and reintegrate with the other two. He describes how small animals have life-threatening experiences from predators all the time and recover quickly, but for us humans, it is the rational brain that blocks the reprocessing. Why?

The energy that is marshalled in a life-threatening or powerfully stressing experience is huge. Think of the mother being able to lift a car off the legs of her child. When neither "fight" nor "flight" are viable options, the body moves into "freeze." Think of the immobility response of the opossum and other prey animals. When we humans start to move out of this frozen state, we are often frightened by the intensity of the energy that needs to be

released, whether it's anger, retribution, shame, judgement, or grief. The rational mind blocks the discharge of these feelings out of the fear that it will be out-of-control, and someone may get hurt. This stalemate becomes a "cold war" between the parts of our brain where the cure and the resolution itself are at odds. The good news is that with proper guidance we can employ simple techniques that are safe and gentle to shake off the trauma of overwhelming events, and unravel the complex mass of symptoms and coping mechanisms.

My friend Dustin is a Vietnam vet and as a young man, went through just about the worst that a war can dish out. For over 25 years, he dealt with the gnawing memories, the depression, and various addictions. Also a massage therapist, he could lose himself by de-stressing others, but hadn't found a way to heal himself of his past experiences of war—until breathwork. He came to six of our seminars and watched the trauma roll off as we introduced incremental openings in his breathing pattern and supported his body's discharge and reorganization. As a healer himself, he knew how to go with it, and trusted his body's process. (You can read his story in the first Stories section in this book.)

Dustin now practices breathwork every day—not for trauma discharge as this has totally left his body—but for oxygenation and detoxing, to stay energized and clear. He is a regular facilitator at our breathwork

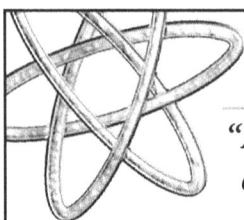

seminars. At a recent check-up at the veteran's hospital, the doctors said he has the biological make-up of a 47-year-old—he's 64. Last month, he did 90 mini-massages all night long at a cancer walk-a-thon. That's his idea of fun.

So trauma is not an incurable disease and its effects (PTSD) don't have to be a "life sentence." Medications can be helpful and necessary in some cases, but drugs involve manipulating and disabling biochemical switches in the body that can hamper the healing on deeper levels. Traditional group or private talk therapies can be lengthy and expensive and "telling the story" can have limited results if real discharge and reintegration are not happening.

Dr. Levine's Somatic Experiencing techniques (visit TraumaHealing.com), and the breathwork approaches of psychotherapist Joy Manné (visit i-Breathe.com) and others, trigger various body changes, called *discharge*, which are key for trauma resolution through body and brain reintegration. These phenomena can include tingling and trembling, spontaneous full-body breathing, body temperature shifts (usually from cold to warm sweating), and can involve emotional release and verbal discharging—all signs that the body's frozen fight-or-flight response is thawing. Levine uses a progressive series of imagined exposures related to the trauma, with a careful watching and managing of the body's "felt sense" reactions. Joy Manné describes her approach with a clients as follows:

"The method I used was to teach him to breathe deeply into his belly and to slow down his breath. I had him place his hands on his belly, one higher than the other so they did not overlap, to increase the area of sensation, and instructed him to breathe "into your hands, so that you can feel your breath caress your palms." When the breath is slow and deeply abdominal, grief [or anger and restimulation] will not get out of control… Once I am convinced that a client is sufficiently grounded and aware for us to start breathwork, all I do is ask

Eye Movement Desensitization and Reprocessing (EMDR)

EMDR is a psychotherapeutic approach developed by Francine Shapiro that uses dual attention stimulation, such as eye movements, bilateral sound, or bilateral tactile stimulation, to resolve symptoms resulting from exposure to a traumatic or distressing event. Clinical trials have demonstrated EMDR's efficacy in the treatment of PTSD. It has shown to be more effective than some alternative treatments and equivalent to cognitive behavioral and exposure therapies. Although some clinicians may use EMDR for various problems, its research support is primarily for disorders stemming from distressing life experiences. ▨

the client. "Put your attention on your breathing and tell me what happens." The client is to give a phenomenological account, describing bodily feelings and breathing rhythms and when they change. Thoughts and ideas are included in this phenomenology. The attention to precision and detail inherent in this technique slows the process and enables dealing with each feeling and sensation as it comes up. Starting like this means that the client is doing a lot of talking in early breathwork sessions and I am doing a lot of listening and responding."[1]

Michael Grant White, creator of Breathing.com, is among the voices cautioning against any high-energy therapy that is aggressive in eliciting cathartic discharge, especially with trauma victims. Some of the early forms of breath-work encouraged high-chest

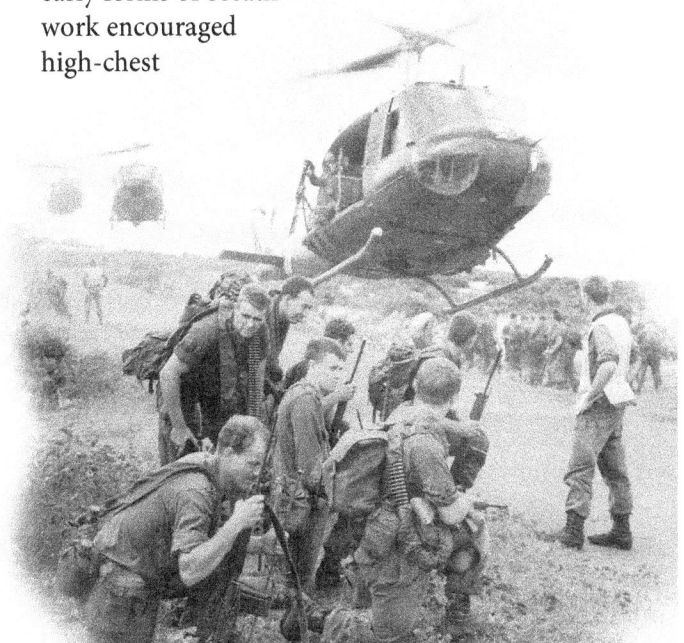

The Hopi Nation

In Anglo-European cultures, it is the needs of the autonomous ego that dominate perception. In the Hopi cultures, it is the needs of the tribal community that are primary.

The Hopi are not alone in this worldview. In many aboriginal cultures, the entire group shares the pain of an injured individual. Because of this felt connection, the healing of a single person naturally becomes the responsibility of the entire group. Specific rituals are performed involving the whole community. The Hopi say that if trauma is not dealt with quickly by the whole group, then its negative consequences will affect the tribe for seven generations.

What happens to cultures whose sole focus is self-involvement and autonomy? What lies in store for countries made up of isolated individuals who have little feeling for being a "people"? They become, as we have, particularly vulnerable to the disconnection that results from traumatic experiences. ■

—Peter A. Levine, Ph.D.

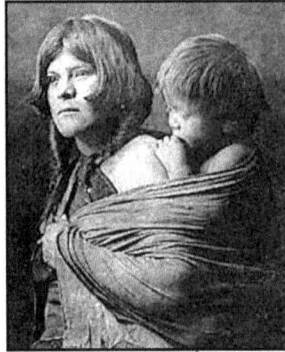

where I believe we should direct everyone for balance, grounding, and accelerated emotional stability. The therapeutic environment should be used for breakthrough work, spiritual principles, practical solutions, and to train, monitor and re-enforce daily breathing practices. I have used mostly gentle techniques and exercises and have purposefully avoided the high-intensity, cathartic styles. I am trained in them and I rarely use them. Inasmuch as the unbalanced breath can result in emotional confusion and overall convoluted energy management, I feel strongly that the professional therapist should know how to develop the breath in the fastest, safest, most grounding, and centering way possible."[2]

Mike White trains therapists at his Optimal Breathing School. He and I have collaborated to develop Integral Breathwork, a bringing together of physiological breathing improvement with transformational breathwork. In the well-worth-reading book, *Body, Breath, & Consciousness*, Drs. Levine and Macnaughton offer the following advice: "Attention to the pattern or type of breathing displayed by a client can provide useful

hyperventilation (rather than gentle diaphragmatic breathing), or paid no attention to breathing-pattern assessment, correction, and improvement before therapy. These approaches can result in "too much coming up too fast" and can retraumatize. A wise saying common among the evolving uses of this therapy is: "You don't push the river!" Here are Mike White's words:

"Self-determinism is almost always the key to lasting results. Daily practice of proper breathing is

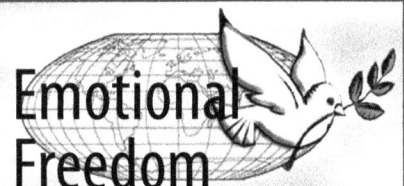

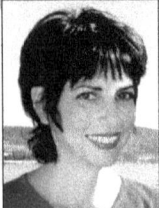

information for the therapist... Intervening in the client's breathing pattern can be useful in moving the client toward self-regulation and a sense of wholeness... Particular cautions need to be kept in mind when there is any evidence of shock or trauma, medical conditions, or dissociative issues."[3]

Now let's look at a few of the other emerging natural approaches to the healing of trauma, some involving neurological reprogramming, others working with the unblocking of energy, such as EMDR, RET and EFT. Still others work with repatterning of beliefs, such as Constellations work and Psych-K. (See sidebars for stories and definitions.)

I spoke recently with another psychiatrist, Dr. S. Robert Martin, himself a Vietnam vet, who has switched from traditional talk therapy, where it typically took 3–4 years of once-a-week sessions to resolve PTSD symptoms, to EMDR therapy, where he is seeing resolution in 3–4 months (for trauma

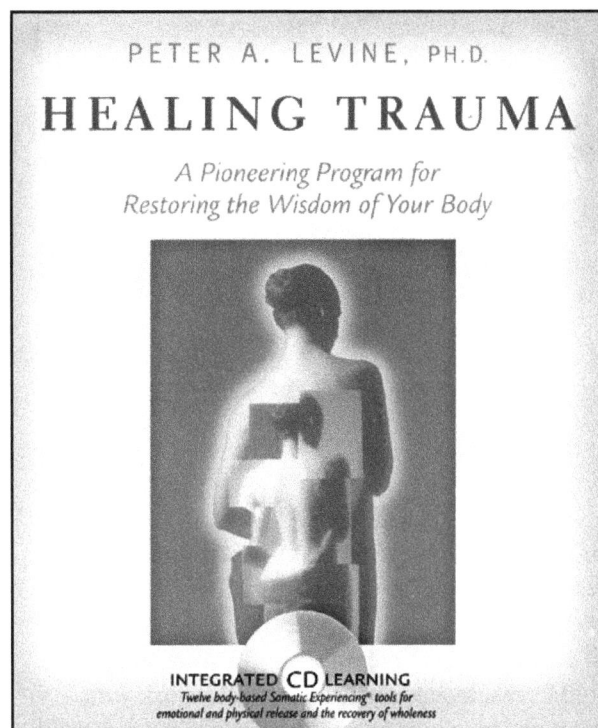

PETER A. LEVINE, PH.D.

HEALING TRAUMA

A Pioneering Program for Restoring the Wisdom of Your Body

INTEGRATED CD LEARNING
Twelve body-based Somatic Experiencing® tools for emotional and physical release and the recovery of wholeness

Psych-K®

We are not born with PTSD, it occurs when something traumatic happens to us. In those moments of trauma, the body and subconscious mind instantaneously develop beliefs that are 'downloaded' into our biological computer. These beliefs, now imprinted on our cells, tend to override all conscious thoughts. We may be unconsciously holding beliefs that tell our body that life is not safe, or that certain persons or animals are a threat. Or, our body/mind may believe that we may be hurt when we go out of the house, or drive a car. Since our subconscious mind is much more powerful than our conscious brain, the beliefs it holds are what determine our personality and our reality. Our biological systems react to what our subconscious mind believes. So when we are in a place that triggers this response, i.e., driving, alone in a dark place, passing a barking dog...our heart rate goes up, it becomes difficult to breathe, we begin to panic and the domino effect kicks in, and we are unable to get to a place that is safe for our body/mind.

In my personal experience using Psych-K to treat PTSD, I did not have to focus on how this all came about. I did not have to know about or restimulate what caused the problem in the first place. I only had to identify what the belief was,

which was easily accomplished with muscle testing. Then, I had to determine what I would prefer instead. For example, I knew that I had a tough time being alone at night, even with the doors locked, the dog next to the bed and a gun in the nightstand. Consciously quite safe, right? Wrong! The panic would kick in and I could not rest until I got up and checked the windows and the doors again, sometimes 10 times a night! So I made a simple statement of, "No matter where I am, I am safe and my body and mind are filled with peace and comfort." Within a few moments of doing this PSYCH-K balance, I noticed a calm come over my body/mind. That night I slept better than I had in years. This has remained the same for over almost 2 years.

I have used this technique on clients who have experienced similar symptoms with various causes. Every time within a few balances, things are noticeably different and have lasting effects, even going so far as to get off of prescription medications (with a physicians' direction). This is a fast, easy, effective way to address the cause, while focusing on the future—focusing on what we want to be true. We are born with a blueprint for wellness, it is the disruptions in this blueprint that cause dysfunction, disorder and disease. It is within each of us to know what we need to heal. ■

Amber Ashby, CSP, CMT
clwd94u@usamontana.com

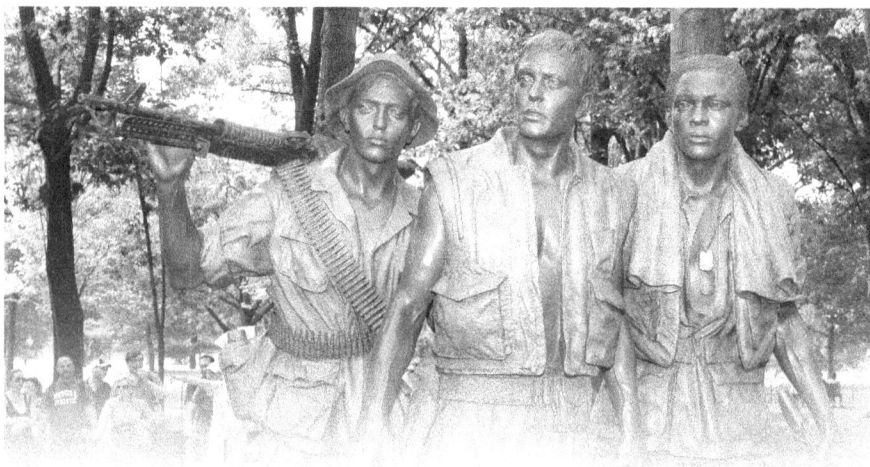

or abuse victims), and even 3–4 sessions for less severe cases (auto accidents). Dr. Martin mentioned that, although EMDR is the treatment of choice by the Veteran's Administration and the Red Cross, he has made attempts to work with veterans' hospitals and insurance companies to get EMDR covered for vets and has met resistance, so for now he sees patients privately. He also introduced me to Dr. Breggin's books (see recommended reading list) on the harmful side effects of drugs for depression and trauma. As you review the stories and descriptions with this article, you'll see that the methods described do not involve a retelling or reliving of the original traumatic experience. (Some will involve discharge and emotional release, while others do not.) In his article, "Nature's Lessons in Healing Trauma," Dr. Levine relates: "I learned that to heal trauma, it was not necessary to dredge up and relive memories. In fact, severe emotional pain can be re-traumatizing. What we need to do to be freed from our symptoms and fears is to arouse our deep physiological resources and consciously utilize them. If we remain ignorant of our power to change the course of our instinctual responses in a proactive rather than reactive way, we will continue being frozen, imprisoned, and in pain.

The tacit acceptance of drugs as the answer to this epidemic is frightening as well as misleading. These so-called disorders are not diseases like pneumonia or juvenile diabetes. Why are we not profoundly disturbed by the creation of future generations of chemically-dependent citizens? Will America become known as the "Prozac nation," unable to function without mood elevators and anti-depressants? Perhaps this situation already exists.

Trauma is about broken connections. Our connections with the body/self, family, friends, community, nature, and spirit have been broken, perpetuating the downward spiral of traumatic dislocation. Healing trauma is about restoring these connections."[4]

Dr. Levine describes trauma as the most avoided, ignored, denied, misunderstood, and untreated cause of human suffering. So many complicated symptoms and maladies arise out of fear as we try to block it. And yet, as I often hear in my seminars, "Could the solution be that simple?" Yes, it can.

As we employ these gentle, natural, and simple modalities, and trust the body's intelligent, self-healing abilities, we can safely overcome the fears that bind us to non-resolution of trauma. Otherwise, the cure itself is at risk of becoming the enemy, and the war within will continue. When portions of the mind/body are disconnected and at odds with each other, when the rational mind won't trust the instincts, where fear, anger, shame, or pain can't resolve, or are chemically suppressed, there will be acting out (violence, abuse), or "acting in" (addictions, self-destructive behavior).

Every man must find his own way to diffuse the tension. *So play with your kids! Get a massage! Go fishin'!* But where there are deeper symptoms of PTSD, seek help, rather than thinking you can just "cowboy up." Men's conditioning and training lead them to either explode or implode when there is too much stored tension and trauma. But what about the women? Well, first off, there are female soldiers too. But most women will end up taking on the suffering of the men they love. Statistics show that up to 80% of all women will be victims of some kind of abuse in their lifetime. It's easier for women to say, "I need help," and easier for them to find their heart and to forgive. So, men, we must first and always protect the ladies in our life from harm. Then in matters of the heart, it's OK to let them lead the way.

Wounded Warriors

by Colin P. Sisson • Excerpts:

[Upon first arriving home from Vietnam in 1967...]

I woke up bathed in sweat, feeling totally disorientated and not knowing where I was. It had been that same nightmare that I had been having every night for over a month... Since those dreams started, they had been getting steadily worse and I was starting to think that I was going crazy...

Mum came up to me and stood behind me, then wrapped her comforting arms around me. "Welcome home, son. I'd like you to know that whatever's going on inside of you, I'm always here for you. You don't have to talk about it. Just know that you are safe at home. I choked back the tears that demanded expression. She cried for me instead, at the same time telling me that, if I wanted to, it was okay to cry too. Her assurance was in vain, for I had a deeply rooted belief that, if I were to survive, I had to keep my feelings under control.

The next day was spent shopping and sightseeing in Auckland. While walking along the street, a car suddenly backfired. The next thing I knew, I was looking out at Mum from underneath another vehicle that was parked. She was staring at me with her head tilted to one side. "Are you all right, son?" I pulled myself from under the car, stood up, and brushed the dust from my jacket. I smiled weakly at her and at several curious passers-by. "Sure, just keeping my reactions in trim," was all I could say. Six months after leaving Vietnam, I was still having nightmares about the war, but by that time I was able to suppress any screams at the point when I woke up. This self-control saved me from having to make embarrassing explanations to my concerned family about the state of my mental health.

[25 years later, Colin is a breathwork trainer...]

In the twenty-five years since my return from Vietnam, I have experienced many radical changes in my life. The most significant was probably, that I gave up my need to regard each potential female partner as a surrogate mother. Secondly, I worked hard at building my self-esteem...

On July 7, 1992, I left New Zealand for Russia, where I had been invited to run a training course for therapists and aspiring practitioners of the technique of Breath Integration. This was my new—and I felt, more appropriate—name for rebirthing. It had been arranged that I would give my services for free, as a contribution to an emerging nation in need of help from the West.

As I came down for breakfast, Eva said, "I think you need to breathe, Colin." Her sharp eyes and intuition missed nothing. "No. I'll be okay in a few hours."

My reply did not fool Eva. "I've known you long enough to know when you are avoiding something important. Come on, I'll 'rebirth' you."

During the next two hours, I exploded with anger and then cried like a wounded baby, digging deeply into my subconscious and discovering emotions I had long forgotten. In the end, I surrendered totally, and felt the joy and the profound relaxation that follows a Breath Integration session. The healing I received related to the battle in operation Coburg, when I had dysentery. In some way, the upcoming training course, even though I was conducting it, had reactivated that memory both mentally and physically, from all those years before.

[At this training, Colin finds that one of his Russian students was among his enemies in Vietnam...]

I was stunned. Suddenly and without warning, I was looking across the room at someone who was my former enemy. Feelings about the war welled up strongly and it was several minutes before I was able to speak. There was neither hostility nor love, only memories. Everyone in the room felt the energy between us as we looked at each other. Neither of us knew what to do with the feelings that were arising, but mercifully, someone rescued the situation by asking a question about an aspect of breathing and its relationship to mental health, and the lessons continued.

Later, the ex-Russian soldier had a breathing session that brought up issues from 25 years earlier in war-torn Vietnam. He exploded angrily, then cried like a hurt child for nearly half an hour. I knew exactly what he was going through, as I had been in a very similar session only days before. Gathering myself, I went over and sat beside him. Then I wrapped him in my arms, held him like a baby, and gently rocked him, feeling the pain slowly leave his body.

Many of the students in the class broke down and openly wept at seeing two former enemies now united as brothers. I was unaware of the commotion in the room, being fully involved with a man whom I could never again hate, for whom I could only feel total love. It was a moving experience for everyone, but no more so than for me and my new Russian brother.

It seemed that I had found why I'd come to Russia: to heal and be healed. Afterwards my new friend hugged me and wept with joy. Then, looking straight at me, he spoke in a torrent of Russian, too fast for me to understand a single word or even for my interpreter to translate. It was not necessary though. The message of love and brotherhood was unmistakable. ▪

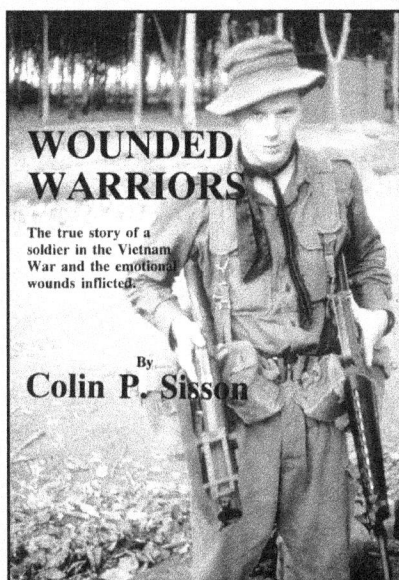

Life-Force Energy (Chi)

Beyond the earth's atmosphere, in what the ancients called the ether, there is an essential substance dispersed throughout space, and everything on earth is designed to attract and retain a certain quantity of this life-bearing substance. Scientists would do well to take up this matter and through laboratory research teach the public about the nature of this quintessence, since it is so necessary to our physical, psychic and spiritual health. The Hindus call this substance prana and have methods for capturing it, particularly by means of the breath. But there are many other methods besides respiration. There is the contemplation of the rising sun and of the starry night sky. There is contact with the forces of nature in the forests, mountains, rivers, lakes and oceans. There is also nutrition, since all the foods we eat contain something of this quintessence, which is distributed everywhere in space, from the rocks to the stars.

Omraam Mikhaël Aïvanhov (1900–1986)
www.Prosveta.com

No discussion of these natural therapies can be complete without an understanding of life-force energy (*chi, prana,* etc.) as all of these methods employ it in one capacity or another. Ultimately, whatever approach to wellness we take, East or West, traditional or alternative, it all comes down to how well and how much this life-force moves through us. Modern medicine is a technical marvel and has saved many lives, and drugs have a valuable place, but they are limited and limiting. A paradigm shift in healing is approaching, along with our view of who we are energetically. Our nature and our potential go way beyond the physical, and even our bodies are way beyond a simple series of biochemical switches. In the meantime, like the Hopi said, "We are our brother's keeper," and we carry each other's burdens collectively.

If you have experienced trauma and are dealing with any PTSD symptoms, there's plenty of hope and help. Seek it. If addictions have set in as coping mechanisms, don't settle for that. You now have the opportunity for probably the most challenging and yet the most rewarding overcoming that we humans can go through. So consider that reward as your grand victory and go for it!

Dr. Levine: "Trauma is about thwarted instincts. Our instinctive energies are not limited to acts of flight or uncontrolled violence. They are our *heroic energies*. And they can be harnessed." Trust in your body's natural healing power! ▪

REFERENCES

1) "Potential Breathwork Specializations: Trauma Treatment," Joy Manné, *The Healing Breath Journal*, Vol. 5, No. 2

2) *Trauflexive* Breathing*, Michael Grant White [*traumas reflected in the breathing], from Breathing.com/articles/trauflexive.htm

3. *Body, Breath, & Consciousness: A Somatics Anthology*, Ian Macnaughton. Chapter: "Breath and Consciousness: Reconsidering the Viability of Breathwork in Psychological and Spiritual Interventions"

4. Article: "Nature's Lessons in Healing Trauma," Dr. Peter A. Levine, at TraumaHealing.com

RECOMMENDED READING

Healing Trauma: A Pioneering Program for Restoring the Wisdom of Your Body, Peter A. Levine, Ph.D. (book & CD; also 6-CD *Sounds True* Learning Course)

Body, Breath, & Consciousness: A Somatics Anthology, Ian Macnaughton

The Body Remembers: The Psychophysiology of Trauma and Trauma Treatment, Babette Rothschild

Soul Therapy, Joy Manné

The Tapping Cure: A Revolutionary System for Rapid Relief from Phobias, Anxiety, Post-Traumatic Stress Disorder and More, Roberta Temes

EMDR: The Breakthrough Therapy for Overcoming Anxiety, Stress, and Trauma, Francine Shapiro

Reclaim Your Light Through the Miracle of Rapid Eye Technology, Ranae Johnson

PSYCH-K: The Missing Peace in Your Life, Robert M. Williams

Wounded Warriors, Colin P. Sisson

Your Drug Might Be Your Problem—How and Why to Stop Taking Psychiatric Medications, Peter R. Breggin, M.D. & David Cohen, Ph.D.

Talking Back To Prozac: What Doctors Aren't Telling You About Today's Most Controversial Drug, Peter R. Breggin, M.D. and Ginger Ross Breggin

Toxic Psychiatry: Why Therapy, Empathy and Love Must Replace the Drugs, Electroshock, and Biochemical Theories of the "New Psychiatry," Peter R. Breggin, M.D.

SYSTEMIC FAMILY CONSTELLATIONS

Systemic Constellations offers an effective way to look at traumatic events from a healing perspective without judgment. Using others to represent the people and issues involved, a healing resolution to the symptoms of PTSD can be found by finally grieving for what happened. The military teaches soldiers how to kill, not how to grieve; and frankly, there's no time for grief in the midst of battle. For civilians, there's no time for grief during war—survival is the only thought. But when there is time, grieving must happen in order to find peace of mind.

If a comrade or relative has died, the survivor may feel guilt that he was not able to save him, or may wish that he would have died too. He also feels anger at the ones who caused the death, which frequently includes anger at God. One way for survivors to resolve their feelings is to know they will live for a while, then they too will die and join the one who died. This gives them permission to live. Since it's only for a while, they can accept life more easily. After a while, if they have been able to grieve, they can accept life and live it fully until it is their natural time to die.

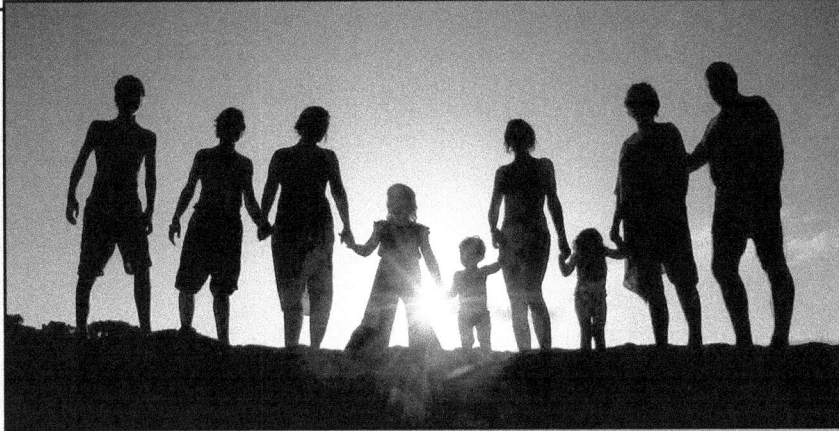

If the trauma was caused by abuse or violence against a person, innocence has been lost and must be grieved for. Soldiers who are severely wounded will be reminded daily of what happened for the rest of their lives, as they live with the consequences. Their anger about the loss of their bodies and lives as they once were must be grieved for, and their new situations must be accepted in order to find peace.

Constellations offer a way to achieve that goal. If a soldier was responsible for the death of an innocent civilian, it is impossible to push that responsibility onto someone else, even if he was a small cog in the military machine. It simply is how it is. When the wrong is acknowledged and faced, when the victim is acknowledged as a person of equal value, respected and mourned, the terrible effects of the wrong can cease.

Peace comes after grieving, after looking at all that has happened, and accepting the fate of those who were affected. Grieving doesn't mean forgetting, which is neither possible nor desirable. It means that as time goes on, the symptoms of PTSD can recede. The constellation process offers you a picture of the solution—a different picture than you currently have. Once your soul has this new picture, it takes over the healing process as it unfolds and is integrated over time, bringing peace back into your life. ■

Visit WisdomHealing.com/wartrauma.htm for more information about war trauma.

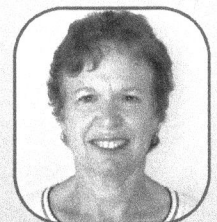

PART TWO

REBIRTHING
according to SPIRIT

Healing with Breath, Light, Sound and Water

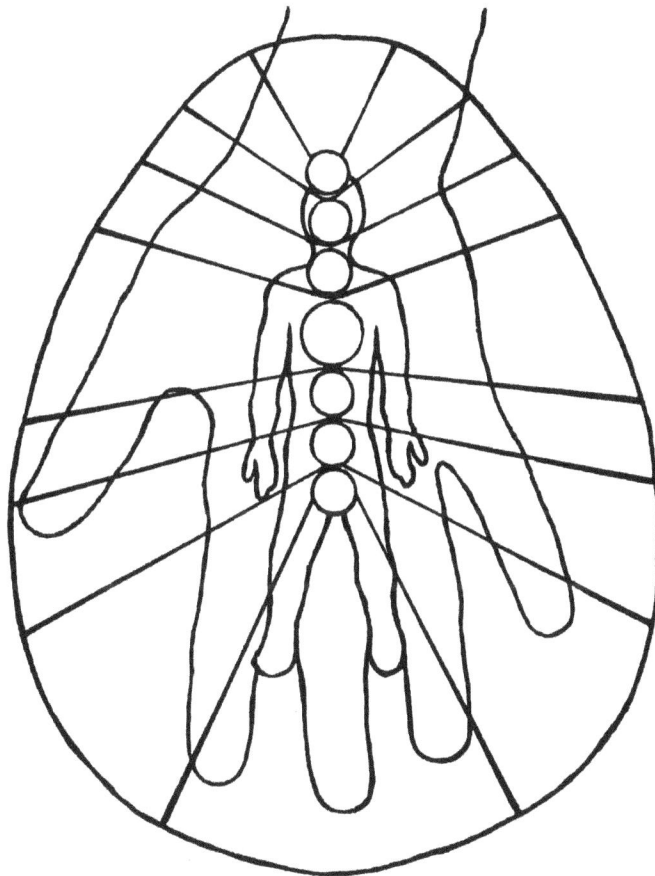

By MOTHER MARY, JOHN THE BAPTIST, JOHN THE DIVINE and others
Through Debra Klein, Michael Richard and Kevin Ryerson
Transcribed and Edited by Denis W. Ouellette

Preface to the 2006 Edition

The teaching manuscripts that form the core of this book were given into my care in the late '70s and early '80s. They have provided a solid basis for my holistic health practice for over 25 years. Long out of print, they are now available to a new generation of breathworkers and to those seeking healing and transformation on all levels. The easy, natural practices outlined in here bridge the gap between ancient rituals and future awakening. They could also bridge the chasm between traditional medical science and natural healing alternatives. In the emerging twenty-first century, quantum physics and medicine are finally embracing the energetic core of our nature. As you will read, the breath and the other elemental forces employed here are effective for healing because they address the whole person— physical, mental, emotional, and energetic. These healing tools are gentle, free, and quite marvelous! Try them for yourself.

THEN AND NOW

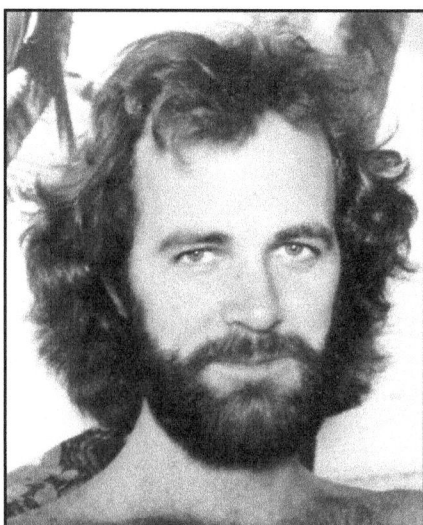

In the early '80s, I was in my late twenties and living in San Diego. Life was good. I was out of the Navy, grew out my hair, and got involved in holistic health and spirituality with a close-knit group of like-minded friends. Back then, San Diego was a mecca for the body-mind-spirit revolution—if anyone was doing it, we were. Rebirthing, the prevailing form of breathwork at the time, was one of the popular healing arts. We launched into it and did a lot of it. We studied with Leonard Orr, Rebirthing's founder, and with Sondra Ray, who led her Loving Relationships Trainings (LRTs).*[1]

I was also working for an herbal tincture maker and herb distributor called The Medicine Wheel. The owners, the Kleins, my good friends, were steeped in Native American lore and teachings. Debra held channeling circles where the famous Apache chief Cochise would speak through her. Also, on occasion, we had visits from Mother Mary. None of this seemed strange to us at the time; this was Southern California and we were idealistic young people, children of the Sixties, looking for growth experiences. We embraced what rang true for us and trusted our inner guidance.

I was doing bodywork and breathwork in private practice at the time. I attended two of Debra's circles and heard Cochise talk about how the breath was used for healing in the ancient healing temples on Atlantis. I transcribed the audio recordings of these sessions, and they became the first part of this trilogy. About a year later, Debra provided me with an audio recording from trance channel Kevin Ryerson containing further instruction on these subjects; that material became the second part of this trilogy. The spirits who spoke through Kevin were John the Divine and a comical Irishman named Tom McPherson. Kevin was made famous as the blind trance channel for Shirley MacLaine, his intuitive abilities highlighted in her bestsellers *Out on a Limb, Dancing in the Light,* and *It's All in the Playing,* which first brought reincarnation and new-age thinking to Hollywood and the masses.[2]

*Notes are added at the end of Part Two.

I was so impressed with the clarity of his materials that I met him and did a private reading with him. With these audiotapes in hand, I knew I had the makings of a solid book on the therapies I was learning so much about.

The final part of the trilogy fell into place after I was well along with the transcribing and editing. Another friend in our group, Michael Richard, also had the ability for spirits to speak through him. Through Michael, the spirits of John the Baptist and Katherine the Healer shared their wisdom on these subjects and outlined a beautiful sacred healing ritual practiced by the ancient Essenes.[3] The ritual they described involves seven people supporting an eighth one in water, using light and herbs to infuse the water, doing breathwork, and intoning the *AUM* in alignment with the chakras. On that evening, I was in the water with six others, holding Michael in the manner described as these teachings came through.

A BODY OF LIGHT

Soon afterward, we did several of these remarkable Essene Rebirths together. [See picture in Notes for Part Two.] I can only describe the feeling as "wearing a body of light." Eventually our merry band of healers went their separate ways. After that period, I never sought information from psychics or departed spirits again, nor do I recommend it as a spiritual path. But sometimes a fortuitous window opens from the other side for a true purpose. That purpose in this instance was to bring this self-healing training to you. I published this manuscript in the early '80s under the title *Rebirthing According to Spirit—Healing through Breath, Light, Sound and Water*. It found its way around the world among breathworkers and healers, and from what I've been told, has had a foundational impact.

Fast-forward 25 years. It's 2006, and I'm in my mid-fifties. A strong impulse has led me to continue this work. Using this transcribed text as one of my guides, I have been doing breathwork seminars and trainings for several years. A while back, a breathworker colleague from Atlanta, John Meneghini [see his breathwork CD in Resources] had asked for a copy of the original book. Since it was out of print, it was time for an updated edition.

"I KNOW HOW TO BREATHE!"

From the text, I knew there was a solid physiological basis for why breathwork was so effective as a healing tool. You can use the breath as a doorway into the autonomic (automatic) nervous system. Through breath, you can repair and maintain your internal systems. You can oxygenate and detox the cells to nourish, purge, and heal holistically.

Some people comment, "I don't need to learn how to breathe—I've been doing it all my life!" They don't realize that their breathing and all internal systems (nerves, heart, lungs, lymph, hormones, digestion, elimination, etc.) are functioning at far less than their full capacity. The good digestion that results from diaphragmatic movement, the good detoxing that comes from an efficient exhale usually don't happen well, which leaves them fatigued and sick. Poor breathing causes or worsens every disease. When you clear the cells through good inhales and exhales, the body begins to heal.

Each of our trillions of cells is a highly intelligent computer. Cellular memories are embedded through accident and injury—mental, emotional, and physical. Long after the incidents have passed, their shadow lingers in the cells, creating behavioral patterns, prejudices, etc. These can also come clean. In *Releasing Vietnam*, you read Dustin's story about how, after having coped with horrendous memories of Vietnam for 35 years, the traumatic stress from those events was finally gone from his system after just six breathwork sessions.

OPTIMAL BREATHING˚ SCIENCE

In 2003, our breathwork seminars were going along well. I was developing new techniques and researching those of others, including Dr. Andrew Weil.[4] I discovered Michael Grant White's Optimal Breathing˚ development web site,[5] containing his life's work on breathing dynamics. Mike and I share the goal of bringing a sound physiological understanding and scientific legitimacy to today's arena of breathwork. Our broader goal is the forthcoming partnership of traditional medicine and alternative natural healing.

I have trained with Mike and collaborated with him to create Integral Breathwork˝, which we believe will set a new world paradigm for healing through the breath. It combines the science of Optimal Breathing development, what we call "fixing the plane," with state-of-the-art transformational breath-work, "flying the plane."

In the summer of 2006, Mike and I will have presented the Integral Breathwork Seminars as a teaching model to health professionals at the International Breathworkers Foundation's 13th Annual Global Inspiration Conference, in Nelson, BC, Canada.

FIX THE PLANE!

In our seminars, we show people about good breathing physiology first. We do assessments, measurements, and exercises for improving breathing mechanics. Are they belly- or chest-breathers—and which is better? How can they get the diaphragm moving better? How can good breathing balance the autonomic nervous system? How can they detect and correct obvious and hidden breathing dysfunction and stimulate the optimal breathing reflex?

FLY THE PLANE!

The second half of our seminar starts with applying new tools for client preparation, breath coaching and goal setting. Then we take flight, drawing from the wealth of knowledge garnered from the world's transformational breathworkers.[6] This involves lying down for a full-hour breathwork session using a recorded breathing pattern and orchestral music. [See Resources for breathing-pattern CD and recommended music list.] We integrate our experience with a feast on fruit and nuts, discussion, and a grounding circle.

The formula works. We know because participants consistently describe how they feel with words like peaceful, content, complete, refreshed, grateful, joyful, and grounded. Some exclaim, "I feel like myself again!" or "This seminar has changed my life." [See flyleaves for additional comments made.]

COMMON SENSE

So, is this book for anyone wanting to heal themselves through breathing and the other elemental forces, or is it for professional therapists? Well, it's good for both! We recommend that anyone new to breathwork attend a seminar or work with a private practitioner first. The book is a primer for grasping the potential of this work. Anyone wishing to assist others therapeutically would do well to study this manual and do a lot of private and group breathwork sessions first, and attend Mike's Optimal Breathing School' for training.

Breathwork heals gently and slowly, like peeling layers off an onion, yet dynamic experiences and dramatic breakthroughs can occur. A lot depends on the intentions and experience of both the participant and the breathworker. The elemental life forces carry an innate intelligence that regulates your experience based on your physiology and your most immediate needs.

As you gain understanding and confidence with the process, you can "get in the cockpit" and navigate it more actively, always trusting in your body's ability to heal itself. In 25 years of breathwork practice, I have not seen it to cause harm; nonetheless, some precautions are advised. The supplemental materials in Part Three offer a commonsense guide to keeping your self-healing safe and measured.

Mike White, Dr. Andrew Weil, and others have cautioned that use of certain high-energy and cathartic forms of breathwork can cause emotional, mental, or physical reactions. They also warn that certain Hindu *pranayama* (specific breathing exercises that we do not use) can release energy and activate the *kundalini* life-force along the spine and in the chakras before one is ready to handle this powerful force properly. Professional support and guidance are needed, especially with someone's first experiences. A lot can "roll off" people in the first several sessions, because many of us are carrying heavy burdens. Compassion, intuition, and a depth of experience are essential qualifications of a breathwork facilitator.

Breathing exercises should not be performed while using machinery or driving an automobile as they may cause drowsiness. During initial breathworks, mild to strong muscle cramping (tetany) can occur in the hands and in other parts of the body as toxins and energy are processed and released. This passes. Instructions are given later in the text for its proper handling.

Always be gentle with yourself and ease up if you get physically or emotionally uncomfortable with any changes you are going through. When healing yourself or facilitating another's healing, the Hippocrates principle applies: "First, do no harm." Trust your feelings and gently discontinue a session if something isn't right. The text and additional materials provide valuable guidelines. Please read it all carefully before beginning any practice.

SAFE AND SOUND

The advice given here is not intended to replace professional medical treatment, especially if you are suffering from a disease. Where the text suggests the usefulness of natural healing in relation to certain illnesses or symptoms, it does so to encourage the reader to explore natural alternatives in addition to medical services.

When carried out as described, these simple practices can be beneficial to your physical, mental, emotional, and spiritual well-being. However, if you have a physical, mental, or emotional illness, a serious breathing condition, recent abdominal or chest surgery, heart problems, or if you are pregnant or taking drugs of any kind, do not perform breathwork without first consulting with a qualified healthcare professional.

We again recommend that you work with a certified or experienced practitioner before embarking on private application of these exercises. Perform these exercises safely, carefully, and advisedly. You can heal yourself with these natural forces—it is their purpose. Combine knowledge with common sense (fix the plane first), and then take courage, enter the cockpit, and...

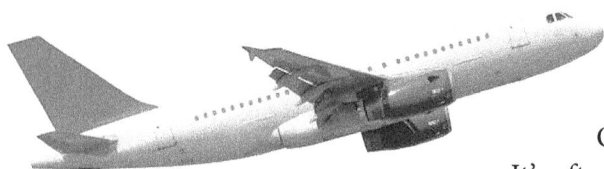

PREPARE FOR TAKEOFF!

Our lives are very full these days—full of stress. It's often enough of a challenge just to get through the day. Breathwork is an important way for people to regroup, find their peace, and "take a breather." At this point, my own breathworks are primarily for maintenance rather than repair. I had dramatic healing sessions along the way, but now breathwork simply refreshes me, fills me with energy and creativity, and prepares me to face my world with gusto.

So what's the goal of all this? Many of us tend to define ourselves by our flaws and our burdened history. Once all this starts to drop away, who will we be? Life's burdens do fall away through this work, replaced with whole-body feelings of peace and joy. You'll be freer to fulfill your highest potential, whatever you can dream that to be. The stuff going into the wastebasket is not the real you, so just let it go. The real you will look better, be more rested, get more done, and have more fun! Remember, energy follows thought. Let your thoughts and energy take flight. Trust the process and enjoy the ride.

You are about to enter a world that may appear to be stranger than fiction complete with Atlantean healing temples and spirits talking to us in everyday language. Parts of this text are as mystical as a dream, parts are densely worded as if from a textbook. Other parts are entertaining and all are enlightening!

If the messenger be an ant, heed it. Yet, as Cochise would say, follow only the truth that feels good to you in your heart. Find that place of intuition within and you'll find your teacher. That voice will heal you. Then you may feel inspired to assist others in their healing.

Namaste—and *Hokahay!*

Denis Ouellette
Emigrant, Montana
March 22, 2006

Introduction to the 1982 Edition

Before you is a trilogy of discourses by six spiritual beings shedding new light on ancient healing therapies. Much of it is about breathwork, a process that uses the breath as a tool for cleansing and integrating the bodies of man—physical, mental, emotional, and the memory. One lies down and breathes in a rhythmic, connected fashion, without pausing between breaths, relaxing on the exhale. This creates and triggers a marvelous energy flow that performs its magic on these many levels.

Between 1979 and 1981, I was present at several of the sessions when these discourses were received telepathically and spoken by the mediums. The communications with beings from higher realms were performed with precaution and sacred intent. The mediums were in a trancelike state.

The presence of the beings was strongly felt during these sessions, and this quality or vibration may again be transmitted as you read the words. You may indeed feel the warmth and peace of Mother Mary, the grand-fatherly presence of Cochise, or the intensity and power of John the Baptist's message. The words themselves, while conveying much learned information, can become the vehicle for an intimate and real energetic communion with these beings.

My work—my pleasure, that is—was to take the audio recordings that were placed in my hands, and give some editorial structure to the informally spoken word while preserving the core teaching and flavor of the originals. Whereas my clairaudient friends served as mouthpieces, I served as arms and legs for our celestial friends who had walked the earth in times past and wanted to share their wisdom and experience on these simple, powerful, and natural forms of self-healing.

Their messages point the way, both in sweeping terms and in practical steps, toward healing ourselves with the help of breath, light, sound, and water—the natural alternatives. This is a manual, not complete but indeed full, for healers to follow and for all those interested in clarity and personal growth.

Before all else, these are spiritual manuscripts that describe all healing as a movement toward God. Healing comes with the realization of, communion with, and surrender to the Eternal Presence that is within and around us. So these words are best suited to those who are ready to bring spirit into their worlds and into the practice of breathwork in particular.

In *Ancient Temple Healing*, Mother Mary comes with blessings and words of comfort, and Cochise opens the Akashic Records[1] to describe Atlantean healing temple practices. In *Self-Healing and Life Extension*, with arcane precision, John the Divine outlines the physiology of breathwork and its application to the chakras; and the jovial Irishman Tom McPherson speaks on the subject of life extension. In *The Essene Rebirth*, Katherine the Healer sets down the guidelines for a powerful form of water breathwork, and John the Baptist delivers a stirring sermon on who we are and why we are here. In addition, Cochise, John the Divine, and Tom answer several direct questions on breathwork and on other fascinating topics that those in attendance were inspired to ask.

With gratitude, we offer to you this gift of knowledge and grace from above.

Denis W. Ouellette
San Diego, California
October 14, 1982

✤—✤ ✤—✤ ✤—✤

ANCIENT HEALING TEMPLE
THROUGH DEBRA KLEIN

BY
MOTHER MARY

AND
COCHISE, CHIEF OF THE
CHIRICAHUA APACHES

✤—✤ ✤—✤ ✤—✤

SAN DIEGO, CALIFORNIA
SEPTEMBER 5 AND 25, 1979

✤—✤ ✤—✤ ✤—✤

MOTHER MARY
You Will Fly to the Stars

Blessings, brothers and sisters! I come on the wings of the dove. My light shines forth onto each one of you. Know that my peace is with you now in your heart. Feel the holy rose of Divine Presence opening up as a flower.

You are flowering inside, each one of you, as you become more and more aware of the radiance and the divinity that you are. Be very aware that you are much more light than you even think at this time. If you were to feel the light that is within you, you could not even handle it at this point. But I see you each as total, realized God-beings. And this is the only thing I see when I look at each one of you. The darkness is but a body, a skin that you wear. And as time goes on, you shed that skin to become more of who you already are.

So for many of you who are in the process of breathwork or other spiritual practices, know that you are not getting any higher, you are just becoming who you already are. And know that, at any instant, all you have to do is recognize the divinity that is within you and you will fly to the stars, out of the bondage of the earth plane, to be one with myself and with Master Jesus and with the many other beings of light who are helping to raise the vibrational frequency of the planet at this time.

My mission is as the comforter—coming to heal, coming to give, coming to love and to help you feel your own inner peace. And so if you feel any pain in your heart, call upon me and I will be with each and every one of you in your time of need. My spirit is in many, many, many places at the same time. My vibration and the vibration of Master Jesus are the yin and the yang, the guardians of this world that hold the earth plane in true light. Many people have seen me, and that is because I appear to them as the comforter on the wings of the dove. And so I go now.

Be aware that breathwork, or the Breath of Life, is a very powerful process, the most powerful process on the earth plane at this time. That is my message. I go now.

Peace be with you!

≫—≪ ≫—≪ ≫—≪

COCHISE
Breathwork's Ancient History

Ho! Greetings tonight to each one of you. Through the waters of your subconscious and into the conscious mind, you have come at this time. And tonight we are gathered to explore a little about that essence of yourself, which has been hidden and buried deep within the subconscious mind, and which has been allowed to come into your consciousness again through the process that is known as breathwork. So I come tonight with many other beings who work specifically with the breathwork process to give you a light onto the subject of breathwork and to look at it from a perspective that is perhaps broader and wider than the perspective that has been given to it in this day and age.

And so it is good to feel the circle and the energy and power of the many beings who are incarnate, those of you in the room right now who have already been working with breathwork. For even with the vibration of the opening that you have allowed yourself to make, the circle is extremely charged and powerful because many of you have allowed yourselves to look at yourselves. And you need to know that among people on the earth plane, that takes great courage. And so this is what I would call and what many in the breathwork process call an acknowledgment. And that is being extended to each one of you here that is actually working with that process, for it takes a lot. It takes a lot when you go out into the world talking and sharing about what you are doing. You will find that many people are not willing to work with this process.

This is a very ancient process. And we are going to talk more about the actual beginnings of this process—where it came from and why it happened and how it happened—when we get more clearly into the trance state.

Know again that there are certain master spirits here tonight. There is one who is called Herakhan Baba[1], whose vibration is present tonight and who is a master of the breathwork process on the planet at this time. There is one who is known as Thoth,[2] who is the vibration of the Atlantean and who is one of the master spirits that brought the whole process of breathwork into knowingness, or into material form. And of course there is the presence of Mother Mary. And there is the presence also of the one who is called Rajneesh[3], the master who, although he does not work specifically with the process of breathwork, works with the processes of letting loose, becoming natural, and getting clear. And so these beings, as well as my own, are here in the circle tonight. Be aware of their love, for the love that encompasses the room now is very strong and very deep indeed.

Know yourselves to be beings of light; and the light that you emanate is love, for the only power in this universe is love. And I come with my heart full of love to give to each one of you tonight and to share that process and that feeling. For I did my process when I did my time, so to speak, on the earth plane.

I feel very good to know that there are such beings around who allow themselves to take themselves into light. For each one of you has a mission that you came upon the planet to do. And you chose to do breathwork even before you came in, because you knew that it would be something that would help you so that you could serve the planet after you had served yourself.

So what I want to do tonight before I go into breathwork any more is to lead you into a meditation that will allow you to become attuned to the process of breathwork and the process of yourselves and the process of this trance circle, to feel this trance circle more. For the trance is a feeling experience. And we want you to experience things, not just hear it on an intellectual level, to get you into a state of trance yourself so that you are absorbing what is said on a subconscious level.

So what I want you to do now is to get into a meditative position, whatever is familiar and comfortable for you. Feel your body relaxing now into that meditative position and begin to watch your breath. Just be aware of yourself breathing in and breathing out in a natural fashion. Do not try to breathe, just be, letting the breath of light and life emanate from within you.

Now visualize a golden light from above coming in through the top of your head in the shape of a pyramid, pouring forth throughout your whole being, cleansing you physically, cleansing you emotionally, and cleansing you psychically. Feel that light permeating every cell in your body. Feel yourself becoming a body of light.

Now, consciously in your own mind, call upon your teachers and guides, whoever they might be. Some of you know and some of you do not know. And now what I want you to do in this state of meditation and light is a simple exercise that many of you already know: staying in a meditative state, doing twenty connected breaths.

[Those present do twenty connected breaths, i.e., smooth and full
rhythmic breaths with no pausing between inhales and exhales.]

What you are doing is allowing yourself to become alive to this process, feeling your body now in a very alive state. You are a body of light. Stay in this state, now, of light. You may stay with your eyes closed or with your eyes open, whatever feels comfortable. And I will continue talking to you about the process that is known as breathwork.

Most people walking on the planet today are walking in a kind of living death. They are not really alive. They have not allowed themselves to be alive since before they were born, and perhaps for countless aeons and aeons of time, as the result of past life. When a soul, when new souls come into materialization on the physical plane, they are quite alive. They are total light. They are total divinity. And they are making their long journey from God to become God.

And so it starts off at a very high level. When people are born into this life after countless lifetimes, some of them will start on a very alive level if their birth trauma is low. There are such beings being born right now through the Leboyer process[4], which is basically natural childbirth with high thoughts and high intentions. And these beings are still as alive and divine and holy as they were when they first left the divine source of creation.

The process of breathwork allows for people to become that newborn soul again. I am not talking about just this lifetime; I am talking about Divinity itself, for each one of you is a divine being. If you knew your magnificence, you wouldn't be able to handle it at this time. For you have what you would call a skin of darkness around you and you just do not know that you are holy and that you are sacred and that you are each Christ yourself.

This process allows for you to realize that and to understand that and to become that again. All that breathwork does is to open you up to who you already are. It is not as if you have to try to go anywhere; you just be. And this process of using the breath allows you to know that aspect of yourself.

Back in the times of Atlantis, when the continents were just being formed on the earth plane, there were beings of light that began the colony known as Lemuria and then, from there, Atlantis. We will speak more of Atlantis and Lemuria at this time. There were many beings who came from other planets and other planes who were beings of light, or what you would call masters at this time. These beings formed the continent of Atlantis and formed the other continents and colonies as well. And when they came onto the earth plane, they knew that the earth had a very special mission to take people through the schools of life. They knew that there had to be a process formed to allow for the beings under their care to know that they are beams, or beings, of light. And so therefore breathwork was developed.

Into the healing temples of Atlantis this process was brought. It was a very sacred undertaking. And in fact, it was used when a candidate came for initiation, which was the process of becoming a master through the raising of vibration. In those times it was very easy to follow steps to become a master. It is a little harder now; you do not just go: A, B, C, and D. For there is no world government as there was then; there is no spiritual link between church and state as there was then. So people would become initiates, and they would become priests and priestesses of the government and of the continent known as Atlantis.

Most people here in this room at this time have had incarnations in Atlantis. Most of you in this room were not of the priesthood. Some of you later on became priests and priestesses in other incarnations, later on in more historical and well-known places, such as Egypt, the Mayan realm, or Tibet. During the time of Atlantis, however, the process of breathwork was developed.

A candidate for initiation used the step-by-step process of breathwork. Breathwork was also used in healing itself. The process of initiation breathwork and the process of healing breathwork were similar but different. A candidate for initiation had seven people present at his or her initiation breathwork, and it was done before the candidate was actually initiated. But I will go on to the basic ideas of what happened.

Before one was to be experiencing the healing, he would spend three days preparing and purifying, using fasting and certain herbal decoctions [or infusions] and light foods. It wasn't total fasting but it was a fast, because any diet that has rules to it can be considered a fast, especially when you are used to eating just about anything. And during this period of time, meditation was used for the person to reflect and to think about what they wanted to get out of this experience. And when the experience took place, the person was totally transformed.

It's a little different now—you have to go through many sessions. But for many people then, one session was all that was needed to be effective to process and work out a particular thing. The preparation took place before the breathwork even happened. The "healee" went through his life and got clear about what he needed for the healing. The initiation candidates went through their whole lives and got clear about what their intentions for initiation were.

In the healing temples of Atlantis were the pools that were used, for they were using water breathwork. If a person was going to be initiated, it was in a very special temple used specifically for initiation. The pool itself was made of red rock, which emanates a positive radiation. White marble was around it. And there was roofing above that allowed the sun to come in, or not be there—whatever was needed. The vibration of the blue ray was charged into the water before the session took place. The way the water was prepared was in such a manner that each new person would have a totally different pool of water. And between sessions they were able to change the water and bring in the vibration of the blue ray within half an hour. For the blue ray is the ray of healing and of truth. Breathwork is a process of learning the truth about yourself.

So the waters were prepared and they were charged with a combination of the blue and the red by laying a blue transparent crystalline substance over the pool and then allowing for the sun to radiate through that crystalline substance into the pool. And this was able to be done, because of the highly evolved technology, within thirty minutes.

The person to be healed came in, and if it was for healing there were two other people present, the principal priest or priestess and the assistant. There were many levels of the priesthood and only the initiates did the breathwork. An initiate was one who had the power of third-eye vision and could see totally what was going on with a person in their breathwork experience.

It is different now because there are not many initiates running around, but there are a lot of people who have been initiated in a prior life or lives who are doing the breathwork at this time. I give you that message. Many of you have not developed that third-eye vision yet, but in a few years more it will be very evident.

And so the person experienced the rebirth. If it was an initiate, there were seven other people in the pool and the pool was large enough for those seven people. Each one represented a certain step of the seven steps of initiation, which correspond to the energy centers, or chakras. There was one person who represented the Godhead, or the seventh level of initiation, who stood at the head of the initiate, and three others on each side who held the person floating in the water as the session took place.

As the person began the breathing process, which is similar to the breathing process used now, whether it was for healing or initiation, special words or mantras were sounded. The vibration of *AUM* was very powerful. The vibration of *THA* was very powerful. And the vibration of *SU* was used as the vibration of allowing for the energies of the emotions, or of what you would call the third chakra, to come out and into the light, for *SU* is light and emotions. Mantras are good now at this time in this age.

I want to update you a little bit on what I am saying, for some of these processes can be used in breathwork now. The three-day fast, which is similar to that of a Native American vision quest and has the same results because you are so clear on what your intentions are, may be used. The charging of the water can be done now in a different way; the people who are familiar with color therapy can tell you about how to do that. And the sacred sounds can be used; it is very powerful and it brings the presence of Spirit into the session immediately. The person in the water hears it and starts getting in touch with Divinity as they are releasing.

What an initiate was doing was allowing the release of all the rest of the "stuff" that was necessary to release before their initiation. And the candidates for priesthood used the process of breathwork more in the healing aspect many, many times before they did what you might call the "grand breathwork."

So the process happened. And while this was going on, an assistant or the breathworker himself would work with crystals in order to draw out certain energies which, through their third eye, they could see needed to be drawn out. The breathworker today could use crystals. But it is important that you have developed a strong trust of your intuitive abilities and a trust of God in order to be a breathworker of high quality and high standards. Only ones who have those standards and qualities and who really know themselves on some level should be allowed to use crystals in breathwork. They are very powerful; for if you have a mind thought that is not of the light (and sometimes it's subconscious and you don't even know about it), it can affect the person that you are working with. Thoughts affect the process whether or not they are magnified by crystals.

Now the session was complete on the level of being in the water with the energy release and the tingling and the getting to feel the divinity. But it wasn't complete on many other levels. There was much more to go, for these temples housed other rooms that the participant was taken into after the session happened.

The priest or priestess who was giving the healing tuned in to the color that the person needed to use to ground out from the session. What you are working with now is called the sealing process. Sealing the session made it so that it did not slip up and so that the person would totally integrate the experience. As many of you know who have done breathwork before, you are not always able to integrate it right away, and it is very important that you give yourself quite a few hours after the session. You do not rush off to do business or to do other things right after. You take time to integrate the process.

And so what happened in these healing temples was that the priest or priestess saw what color of light the person needed to allow for more integration of the experience. And they had the person go in and lie upon a table (similar to a massage table) underneath a ray of light, be it blue or green, red for life energy, pink for love, different rays and different vibrations, whatever was needed. The person lay under that light, called the crystal transformer, which was a direct reflection of the sun through a crystal and which allowed for the experience of that light. The person stayed in this light for the amount of time that was indicated by the priest or priestess, who was able to tune in immediately and who had total third-eye vision and conscious awareness of the Akashic Records and karmic patterns of that person.

Then they went into another tub of water that had special herbs in it. The herbs of myrrh, frankincense, aloe, and cassia, as well as a very nice flower preparation, are good ones to use now and were used in ancient Egypt. There were different herbs in Atlantis, different plant substances. These plants were in the water, like what you would call an herbal bath. And all the toxins that had come out during the session or the light therapy were able to ground out in this water by the pulling action of these herbs, some of which are very astringent and some of which allowed for that person to feel what is called the grounding out and completion process.

And then it was done. And the person was then ready to go on to their initiation or, if it was for healing, to experience what it was like to be reborn. Sometimes breathwork was used in combination with regressive hypnosis. Among the Essenes this was done very strongly, and it will be spoken of in a little bit.

I wish to let you know that, that which is called breathwork is the most powerful process on the planet today for getting you clear. Because what breathwork does is open you up, but it doesn't get you out of balance in the process, as a sudden rush of kundalini would, because it keeps you in your body at the same time. Too often people open up spiritually and psychically but they are not able to do what is the basic, which is having their feet on the ground and their head in the sky. And sometimes during the process, especially in the beginning, you experience a little bit of ungroundedness. But with a few grounding exercises and some extra time, you are basically able to stay grounded.

Regression is also a powerful therapy and I would suggest that sometimes you combine breathwork with regression. And sometimes you'll find yourself regressing anyway in breathwork. What I want to say to you is this: I have a feeling that past lives have more responsibility than some would say. But I am speaking to you as one who reads the Akashic Records and knows where things go. The problem is that people get too caught up in the ego aspects of past lives. But you may use them to develop and open yourself up to the talents that are already inherent within you.

So I wish to go now and allow for the one who calls herself the World Mother to speak to you. I will be back to answer questions.

＊—＊　＊—＊　＊—＊

MOTHER MARY
Essene Breathwork Practices

Blessings! On the wings of the white dove I come to pour onto you love and the light of the Christ that is within each one of your hearts. Know yourselves to be the Sons and Daughters of God. Know yourselves to be divine. For as I come, I see only divinity. I see only the light that is within each one of you. I do not see the darkness that many of you are peering out through—and many of you know yourselves to have these traits of darkness within you.

And so I come tonight to share with you perceptions of that practice that is known as the Breath of Life, the process that was practiced by the Essenes, a Hebrew sect, thousands of years ago, even before the Master Jesus came onto this planet. As a young maiden, I myself experienced the Breath of Life and worked with this process, for my parents were ones who were involved in the spiritual teachings of the Essenes. They were very high in their energy and worked in the healing practices of what you would call the inner circle of the Essenes. I do not wish to go too much into that at this time. But I do mention that I was conceived in a fashion similar to the Master Jesus, and among the inner circle there was what is known as celibacy.

And so my message tonight is that of the workings of the Breath of Life. Each one of you is familiar with that process on some level. And I do not wish to go too much into the actual workings, but to say that it was practiced in that which is known as the Dead Sea and also in the mineral springs in that area, and the region now known as Israel and the Holy Land.

It was used with sacred chants similar to what Cochise mentioned were used in Atlantis, for it was brought to the Hebraic race and to the Essenes from Egypt, and it was brought to Egypt from Atlantis. It was used in combination with hypnosis to take the person into a healing state, and there were many who did the work with the healee. The chants, the actual breathwork, and the sealing process were used among the Essenes. As far as details go, it is not my work to share this at this time; the one who is called Cochise gives far better explanation.

I only wish to say to you, know yourselves. And allow yourselves to open up each day more and more to that light within you. I come as the comforter and the World Mother to give you each peace and love and feelings of divinity and devotion. Know yourselves to be Christ right now. Know yourselves to be light right now. And know yourselves to be divine. For I come and you associate me with divinity, but each one of you is as divine and holy as I am.

And so in love and on the wings of the dove of peace, I go. Feel my love in your hearts now and know that I am with you. Call on me during your healing. Call on me whenever you wish.

Peace be unto you!

❧—❦ ❧—❦ ❧—❦

COCHISE
Native American Medicine

I be back. And I have message to give before we go into questions. Hold on one moment...sometimes hard to come back into *yang* vibration after extreme *yin*...Okay.

Message I give is from certain American Indian tribes who have used the process of breathwork. The message is this: What they worked with among the different tribes was a similar process in the hot sulphur springs around the country. They did not use the process of the breathing as strongly as people use it now, but what they worked with was the water. And they worked with the Grandmother Moon, which is the energy of the vibration of intuition, the moon representing the deepness of Spirit and the deepness of the water.

And so the medicine people or the shamans would do chants over the one who was experiencing this healing, or baptism, or whatever you want to call it. It was a process used for healing, similar to what was used in the sweat lodges, in order to purify and to clear and to get the person into a certain state of consciousness in order to do medicine.

So that is what it was used for—to allow for the practice of medicine. And it was not done as much with the breathing, although every once in a while one would go into a spontaneous breath release. But basically it was worked more with the invoking of the presence and energy of Grandmother Moon. Certain power objects were used. And the medicine people who had direct contact with that energy, for whom the moon was their medicine energy, their medicine way, would work with that person in the process of healing. Among the Warm Springs Apaches this was used. And among other tribes up near the Great Lakes this was used. And among different tribes through America, this was used in different ways. It was a process and it was very strong, but it was used mainly in conjunction with the practice of medicine.

So that is my message at this time as to the workings of breathwork among the Indian tribes. It has also been used by many other cultures and in many different ways. It has happened among the Japanese who have worked with the warm baths. It has happened among many others, but I do not wish to go into that, for we could be here all night.

So I will answer questions now, but first I would like to give you a little bit of information and clarification about working with questions. What happens is you will ask questions and I will give you guidance. I will be reading from the Akashic Records or from your higher selves or from what comes to me through my teachers.

And if the answer feels good in your heart, that is good—follow your heart. If it does not feel good to your heart, if it does not feel right—follow your heart. For I am only a guide. I am only one who comes to serve you. And it is very important, when you are talking about spiritual matters, that free will always be exercised. And if there is not free will, if you come across a teacher who says you should do this or you shouldn't do that, then that being is not working with the highest spiritual principles or with the light. And I would suggest you find somebody else who always gives you that free will, who is not laying their trip (so to speak in modern terms) upon you.

So I only come as a guide and my answers are only given from what I see. And I have perhaps a little more perception because I am working on the spirit level. Follow your heart always in every question that is answered for you. My work is as the humble servant, as is the trance channel whom I am speaking through.

QUESTIONS & ANSWERS BY COCHISE

Arthur: Yes, could you...?

Greetings to you tonight, Arthur. It is good to feel your presence. I have been around you a little more than you think. So have been a few others. There be one called Herakhan Baba who be whirling about you right now.

Arthur: I really don't tune in to those vibrations a lot during the day.

Believe it or not, they are loading you with all kinds of impressions which you are not always allowing yourself to feel. So my suggestion to you is to open yourself up. At least three times a day, sit down and still yourself and say, "I want to be open, I want to receive." Take about twenty connected breaths and then see what happens. That be my suggestion to you.

1. Thank you. I was wondering if you could say anything about womb consciousness, if there are any ill effects that we have from when we were hanging out in the womb the first nine months?

A lot depends on what your parents were thinking at the time. It isn't only womb consciousness, it's what happened when you were conceived. If you were conceived in a violent way, you will experience, even before you become a physical entity, the feelings of violence. And when you are born you will most likely be born in a violent manner because the karma has already perpetuated itself and your thought forms are that the world out there is violent. If the parents were in a place of indecision, if perhaps the mother wanted to have an abortion, the child will feel that and recognize it and they may experience the feeling that their momma was not there for them, their mother was going to leave them. And then later on as they are growing up they always feel that their mother is going to leave them.

But if your parents are coming from a loving place, you will experience acceptance. That does not mean that they have to be godlike, since human nature is such that people tend not to be loving all the time. So you can experience good and bad things in the womb. When you're in there it is a very pleasant environment. And what happens is that when you start getting pushed, so to speak, when the contractions start happening, an incredible amount of fear and adrenaline comes up in a being who does not feel good about what the outside world has to offer. And there begins this incredible struggle and battle where the being says, "I do not want to be born." And so sometimes a long labor will result, which is a trauma for the mother and the child. And if the mother is resisting the birth, then there is more trauma that is inflicted upon the child. And so hanging out in the womb is a good place, but hearing about what's going on outside there can be very scary. Do you understand what I am saying?

2. I notice that a person goes through certain stages in getting clear through breathwork. For example, they may go through letting go of fear and sadness and then they begin to release their breath automatically and their breath becomes fuller. I was wondering if there is a pattern that you could talk about, or certain plateaus.

It would be similar to what you would call the seven levels of initiation. And without going into it in full detail, what I can say is the process does not end until you are fully enlightened. So you will continue to process and process for a long period of time. After you have had your breath releases, it does not mean that you are going to be forever clear. You will have clear periods and periods when more stuff is ready to come up. At a point after the initial six to ten or twelve sessions, the major cleansing is complete and you begin another kind of process, which takes a little more time.

You need to embark on a spiritual path at that time in accordance with your own personal karma and your own personal way. Because, again, it is taking you into the light—toward God, toward total letting go of all earthly bondage, and toward mastery of the earth plane. Do you understand?

3. I've had a vision for many years about a place of purification such as you mentioned with the halls and the baths, like a temple. Does such a place exist and, if not, do we need to create it?

On the etheric it definitely exists, but on the physical it has not been built in this day. There are a couple of groups in this country who have a similar vision. However, to follow it out in the aspect of an Atlantean or Egyptian temple, nobody has yet had that vision. This could be very powerful, but the ones working with it would have to share a common vision and not deviate into all these different paths.

I wish to say that it is good where these sanctuaries are happening where there are so many different paths that are followed. Everybody has a different spiritual path they're on. But sometimes that makes for the meditation space and the healing space to not be as focused. They are universal and that is good; I think that is very important.

But at the same time there is also a need for centers that can fine-tune and focus upon a certain aspect. The opportunities are there, but I make a warning to anyone who plans to carry out an Atlantean/Egyptian type of healing center. They will have to stay on a very high vibrational frequency to work with those powers. And as you are working with initiation, one working in such a center will have to be very committed, whether a total initiate or very close. It is very important that this be so.

4. Could you speak to us about the role of sexuality in the process of enlightenment, about the use of the sexual energy or the kundalini energy?

I say this to you: You can work together in a relationship only so far. Priests and priestesses could have concourse—that is the word that was used—but you need to realize that the path to God is through oneself, totally going into the space of one's aloneness and surrender to God. For the true sexuality or the true tantric marriage is between the initiate and the Father or the Creator.

You can use the tantric energy to bring yourself into a place of visions, good dreams and high spiritual energy and even a mergence with the Creator. But when that happens, it is still your journey. For never on the physical can you totally merge with a person. You can merge with a person, but in the long run it's your spirits that will be merging. And when your spirits become one, you will become one with the Great Spirit, the Creator.

But the final journey, when you actually take it, has to be done alone. And so it is important, when one is in a relationship and both partners are on the path, that a time be set apart in spiritual work as well as other work.

Working together in a tantric relationship on a spiritual path is very powerful. For what you do is you take each other through many initiations and tests. A lot of work with a partner is that of clearing and also using the power and the energy of the opposites, the yin and the yang, to go into places of divine energy, to feel the divine energy.

But it always has to be balanced out. For if you were to get caught up in the relationship and become attached—as people can get attached to tantra—and then the tantric partner leaves, where are you? Ready for another attachment? Do you see what I am saying? In the long run the sexuality is good, but it is important that it be used in a very sacred way.

5. At what point can a person do breathwork on himself and get full value from it, or does one need a breathworker even after several sessions?

Definitely by another person even after many times, yes. You can do breathwork on yourself but it is still good to have a guide. I would suggest, however, that when you yourself reach a certain level, the breathworker you choose is, himself, one who has a very high level of clearance. As when we spoke of the priests and priestesses, you want to look for someone with third-eye vision or at least a very good intuitive sense who can help you past the blocks where you are perhaps stuck. Having someone who is very clear will allow you to go deep enough to process those blocked areas. Also, you may want to combine this with forms of regression therapy, going back to that stuck place and releasing that blockage.

6. Cochise, would you tell us a little about the future of breathwork?

Ho! ho! Need to crack a few jokes every once in a while; it gets too serious in here sometimes…. Remember, laughter is the joy of God, laughter is the light of God. God likes to see happiness, for the abundance of spirit is true joy. The abundance of divinity is feeling your own light.

And so the answer to your question is that it can go everywhere; it is an unlimited process. And many of the processes that we have spoken of tonight can be revived and used in many different ways. The way the process is worked with now through the Theta organization* is very good, because the public needs to be educated about breathwork;

---

*The Theta House, started in San Francisco in 1974, was the first rebirthing/breathwork center.

and some of these methods I have mentioned may seem to be a little too, oh, "occultish" or something. But it may be combined with massage, color therapy, crystal therapy, and hypnosis. [See *Young Indian Brave* in More Stories.] And there is more and more.

7. Would you say something about the use of sacramental herbs and the psychotropic plants and their use in breathwork?

Figures you would ask that question! [This question was asked by Debra Klein's husband, a student of Native American medicine.] This one over here is real good at that. Message to you… I be joking, of course; you understand that I have answered that question already in another trance. But I will say to you this: It is very, very important that if you are doing it you work with one who knows those plants well, has somewhat of a third-eye vision or intuition, someone whom you would trust your life with (I'm talking about the breath-worker now), and that you make a very wise decision. I would suggest the breathworker be partly responsible for the decision; and I do not suggest that many people work with it, only ones who are very comfortable in having used the plants before. But it is not something I would even talk much about to the mass of people. It is something that is for only very special usage, because you want to be careful that there is nothing that happens that is out of control. Do you understand what I am saying?

I again give a stern warning in the use of psychotropic plants in conjunction with breathwork.

8. Can you think of one thing that can be said to someone to encourage them to get involved or to continue with breathwork? Is there one focal thing that people are really interested in?

Hold on one moment…. "If you want to be happy, you need to know yourself." The key phrase is "know thyself." That is one that has been used many times; it is a catch-all to many people. When bringing it forth, mention knowing yourself and also mention how most people go around in a fog, in a daze. In your breathwork seminars, what you might want to do is an exercise with people that would show them how unaware they are in their daily lives and what happens to them. And then share with them an experience of what it's like to be conscious, perhaps by doing twenty connected breaths. Show them what it's like to feel. There are many things you can do to get people interested. Basically you want to give people an experiential knowledge of the possibilities and value of working in this process.

9. **Do you think doing twenty connected breaths is enough for people to get that experience?**

It depends. What can be very powerful is when you pair up with another person and do twenty connected breaths together. Or do the light meditation similar to what we did earlier. A nice way to start a breathwork seminar is with a little meditation. It doesn't have to be called that, because you might get some people confused about it or who would feel, "Oh, meditation, that's religious." What you might say is, "Let's do an exercise," or a "process," if you will.

10. **I have a question about resistance. You find someone who thinks they are doomed for failure and they keep falling asleep in their sessions. Would it be better to sometimes just let them fall asleep?**

Each breathworker makes his own decision on that. It would be best to feel the flow as it is going. There are some people that you have to shake up or else they won't do anything. Either by continuing to wake them up or by doing some of the processes that are actual manipulations of the chakras, you get them to release that block that is knocking them out. A person will not go to sleep if he is feeling somebody pressing a pressure point that does not feel too comfortable, like the points at the feet. And the pressure points will sometimes activate that person so much that he will deal and move with it. You have to follow your intuition.

Again, that is the most important requirement of a breathworker. One who has an intuitive knowledge of what is going on in the session will be inspired to do the right thing. Follow that inner voice, that psychic impressional input that tells you what to do. If you follow the first thought that comes into your mind, you will most likely be right. All psychic input is usually essentially correct; it's just that you start to rationalize it and invite your mind along to the party, so to speak.

Debra's husband: Sounds like Rajneesh coming through.

Debra be smiling through the trance. There be one by the name of Denis here?

Denis: Denis here!

You like to joke too; that be good. Message to you be: You be good transcriber. I wish to give you message that you be doing good work. You know vibrations of Cochise well. I like your transcribing and it helps to raise your consciousness to do it. And I be with you sometimes when be sitting there grinding away at it. That be added benefit.

There be others in the room right now; however, I am not given permission to go on. I have what is called the Lords of Karma working with me who tell me what to say and who to say things to. There be others that I send you my silent love and my presence. Feel my presence within you now, and know that the light that I give and that I have comes to you with total love and total clarity.

And so I am going to go now and wish to let you all know that you are special. Tell the people around you about this process. And know yourselves to be Sons and Daughters of God, ones who carry the light within your heart. And know that, as Jesus said in the Bible, "You shall do greater things," you are doing them, just by the very process of becoming clear and becoming one with your Divine Spirit.

And so in love and in truth and in light, and in the spirit of Christ Consciousness, I go now. *Hokahay!*

❖——❖ ❖——❖ ❖——❖

❦——❦ ❦——❦ ❦——❦

SELF-HEALING & LIFE EXTENSION
THROUGH KEVIN RYERSON

BY
JOHN THE DIVINE

AND
TOM McPHERSON

❦——❦ ❦——❦ ❦——❦

SAN DIEGO, CALIFORNIA
SEPTEMBER 19, 1980

❦——❦ ❦——❦ ❦——❦

JOHN THE DIVINE
Physiology of Breathwork & Chakra Work

We would like to receive information about breathwork that would be useful to us as a learning group and in our practices with others.

You will find that breathwork, as brought forth in the West, is a technique used to facilitate a connection within various structures of the psychology for the return of the consciousness to the levels of the womb—a technique wherein there is the regression and the putting to rest of the conscious mind, creating the ability to tap into various other levels of psychic force within the mind. You will find that breathwork has been used in many cultures, predominantly in India and through areas of China, dating back to Atlantis and Lemuria.

As to the technique itself, it will be found as the use of the rhythmatic breath, which stimulates a specific state of metabolism within the body that identifies and duplicates upon many other levels as well. This state affects not only the complete oxygenation of the body and release of carbon dioxide, but more so an actual stimulation of the metabolism, triggered as an altered state, allowing the conscious mind to extend itself into the physical form, for the physical body is actually itself a manifestation of the subconscious and conscious mind. This is why there are often generally observed in breathwork such activities as the cramping of the muscular tissues, since the cellular memories of the muscular tissues themselves become activated. [See *Tetany & Gentle Breathwork* in Articles.] Even as you have identified in various other body-mind techniques, the muscular tissues are critical in the storage not only of cellular memories but of the subconscious mind faculties as well. Thus breathwork in the first level or phase deals with the cleansing of stored memories from the current lifetime and those states proceeding to the altered states of the subconscious faculties.

But once there is the putting to rest, more so the putting, as into an ordered priority, the current levels of emotional qualities of the individual, including the conditionings from childhood proceeding from parental lineage, interdynamics with siblings, and personal transformations and survival needs of the body physical, then there can be the actualization of the spiritual self. For while breathwork has been used in the context of a body-mind principle, advancements in the community of the holistic-health fields are incorporating more so now the concept of the totality of self—body, mind, and spirit. Spirit here represents in its fullest context the forces of the soul itself. Therefore, the use of breathwork has been extended to the treatment of past lives, aligning the psychological principles of past lives as they apply to the actualization of the ability to function with greater clarity in supplying the emotional needs of the current psychological self.

You will find, as to the next current extension of breathwork as a tool, that there will be the ability to draw into the self not only the rudimentary psychic faculties activating the abilities of prognostic experience, abilities to have intuitive memories of the past, or the increase of the telepathic abilities—more so there should be the development so as to bring about divine psychology into this system of therapy, bringing about the Christ Principle itself into activation.

When breathwork is applied to specific areas within the physical form, these would be found to be working within the activities of the chakric areas. For once the individual has been stimulated past the traditional forms of breathwork, be this in the dry or as in the use of the waters, then the conscious self has been properly prepared in its own right to extend itself into the soul's forces. These early phases are, again, for aligning the current psychology and emotional needs and for bringing clarity to the functioning conscious self.

When there is the triggering of these activities, breathwork, through connected breath and even through visualization and other forms of the current practice, could then come into a diamond focus specifically with each chakra, or seat of consciousness. The use of breathwork as channel to the seven chakric modes would be as follows:

The primary seat of consciousness within the base chakra is found within the context of the coccyx. This is, of course, at the base of the spine within the conical tissues known as the sacrum. The secondary level of the chakric seats of consciousness is known as the sexual chakra, which in males is found in the testicles and in the females, the ovaries. The third level is found within the abdomen—the stomach or solar plexus area. Then you would find the fourth level contained both within the thymus and the organ of the concentration of muscular tissues known as the heart. The fifth level is within the thyroid as well as the parasympathetic ganglion stored in the neurological tissues within the spinal column. Then, sixth and seventh are found within the two master glands of the pituitary and the pineal, centered at the third eye and within the skull.

Breathwork as used in connection with these specific areas has the advantage of activating two forces, twofold. These are the seats of consciousness of the Spirit, which resides within ye as a soul firstly, and then there are involved the electromagnetic and neurological energies. But above all, there can be the activation of physiological processes within the body physical for transformation of a very specialized degree. For when you are attempting to bring about the state in breathwork of the level of consciousness associated with the context of the womb, you will find that you are also stimulating the metabolism on a physical level. The conscious mind is regressing itself to that higher level of cellular development when it overshadows the body physical, duplicating the metabolism of the embryo and re-creating that heightened faculty.

This reactivates the most sensitive activities within the metabolism and the greatest point of growth in activity within the body physical so as to allow an impression and an activation of the seat of consciousness. That is, when there is the conscious extension backwards through the cellular memories to the point of experiencing birth in the womb, you will find that the metabolism is also duplicating the actual cellular activities and enzymatic activities in stimulation directly also to the molecular levels of that which was inhabited within the time period of the development of the embryo itself, particularly after the first four critical months when the soul overshadows these activities.

Then, when the conscious mind has attained that level of altered state through the guidance of the breathworker, or when engaged in breathwork by oneself, focus may be guided to the channeling of energy into each of the chakric centers for the revitalization and actual rebuilding of the balance within the contexts of each center. And again, this activity is not only to activate that seat of consciousness upon the level of the spiritual forces dwelling therein, but also the physiological processes in each, since the physical itself is stimulated through those sensitive psychological responses.

You will find, for instance, that the base chakra is associated with actualizing personality, that it would draw in specific past-life forces providing the individual with the ability to remain in the grounded aspect of the practical functioning personality. This is the ability of relating to others yet still maintaining the identity of self—remaining the grounded being without wandering into various other forms and levels. Past lives, for instance, wherein the individual demonstrated authority and strength or the ability to negotiate for needs of self and others, would be drawn in to strengthen self. But also there would be the stimulation of the physiological processes so as to remove fears and other ungrounding principles.

For you will find that the coccyx is a critical reflex point in the body where both spiritual and neurological energies are concentrated. Through concentration of the breath and awareness here, there is a direct stimulation and balance of the adrenal, or supra-renal, glands. Underactivity of the adrenals manifests incompetence within self. So therefore, directing and concentrating the energy in this way balances the creative forces within self by either stimulation or de-stimulation of the adrenals. The mind, through the process of breathwork, becomes the architect both spiritually and physiologically from that existence in the altered state.

The secondary level would be the sexual chakra, wherein lies the raw creative force. The sexual chakras, both within men and women, are in critical relation with the levels of protein in the body. It will be noted that when there is the stimulation of added protein within the system, the individual may become as the creative or overly aggressive being. Also, when there is the lack of protein, too much of the pacifist is observed.

In studying the patterns of the low- and high-protein diets, it is noted that those who take high quantities of meat, or approximately 75 grams of protein into the system, exhibit more so the elements of imbalance. Those who take from 25 to 36 grams of protein approach more so the correct balance. Those who take only 10 to 15 grams of protein are the overly passive types with lack of stimulation and creative abilities, unless these are offset through the fruitarian diet pattern wherein the blood sugars overtake these programmings.

Within the average individual, the proper balance of protein intake, along with the critical digestive enzymes from vegetable sources for assimilation of foodstuffs and nutrients, has primary impact upon the creative course of both the metabolic and biological personality. Also, aspects of sexuality classically associated with this chakra, as in tantric practices from Atlantis, India, or China, and difficulties or imbalances obtained from past lives may be addressed here both spiritually and physiologically as they portray in influencing the creative and motivative forces.

The third chakra is of the emotions. Emotionality is incorrect; sensitivity is the correct balance here. Sensitivity is as in the ability to listen and feel with thine own emotions. The balancing of this chakra lies in the obtainment of knowledge of one's own emotional imbalances. It is noted that the partaking of foodstuffs is directly associated with the stomach. Overly emotional people will oftentimes have an excess of fatty tissue in this area so as to insulate themselves from the feeling of emotions. This is often associated with the lowering of self-esteem and a lack of feelings or emotions, quite often as associated with the parental images. The proper metabolism and, again, past lives associated with the emotions are brought to balance through this chakra.

The heart chakra is the great balancer, balancing all the four lower chakras. The fourth chakra is of course the love center, which brings about the ability for the personal expression of the Greater Self.

The thyroid itself is critical to the bringing forth of balance to the muscular tissues and metabolism as a whole. The throat chakra then will bring about greater confidence in self as well as the abilities of self-expression.

The pituitary is in association with a personal relationship with God. It brings forth the stimulation of various natural hallucinogenics identified as the visionary qualities of the third-eye chakra and is also critical in stimulating the dream state.

Within the capacity of the pineal gland lies the interconnectedness with the higher forces and the abilities to merge with same. The crown chakra is for the focus of the consciousness of God, wherein access is gained to all knowingness and wisdom.

Working with these seats of consciousness, then, to actualize the self in a conscious and knowledgeable manner, rather than in a haphazard or spontaneous manner, gives to the discipline of breathwork a greater measure of control. Interrelating these with the technique of connected breath as stimulation to bring about the altered state as in the womb, sensitizing the body again to those forces of embryonic metabolism and indeed as an extension of the body's own natural biofeedback system, we then work with the chakric system.

For instance, if it is noted with the individual that there is an ungroundedness, immediately go to the base chakra. For difficulties in sexuality, visualization and focus of breath in the second chakra is wise. To obtain betterment of results with the first three chakras, it would be suggested to apply a quickening of the breath to bring about the theta state of altered awareness. Then, as to the heart center, more so a regular rhythmatic breath is recommended since this is closer to the lung center itself. With the higher centers, the theta state may be contacted through a deeper, more passive system of breath. Each of these may be personalized to the individual.

This system or spectrum of breathing rhythmatics, working in conjunction with the chakra centers, is indeed a wise pursuit. For you will find that the breath is the only autonomic function within the body physical over which the individual may esteem conscious control. Thus rhythmatics, or the connected breath, is the key to the body being the anchor in consciousness for the soul's forces on this plane. By its being both an autonomic and yet a conscious voluntary response, the breath, concentrated again to the actualization process with the seven chakras mentioned, becomes the bridge between the sympathetic, parasympathetic, and autonomic nervous systems and the link between the conscious, subconscious, and superconscious selves.

Studies, then, in brief review of results desired in breathwork would be, first, obtainment of the state familiar as the regression to the womb, brought about almost spontaneously by the activation through connected breath of the cellular memories. This is where the soul's forces meet the body physical, particularly a stretching back to the existence of the embryonic state of the fourth month. For this is the point of the incarnation of the soul into the body physical. There can then be the duplication through consciousness of the sensitivity to that state of metabolism, putting ye in fully conscious attunement with the soul's forces in their original and purest state.

These techniques under the guidance of the breathworker would be wiser to pursue in the waters rather than as in dry breathwork. For the waters—particularly those in a state of fluid motion, still purer when with an element of mineral content—constantly cleanse the aura of any subconscious negativity as this is released. The modern technologies of heated and swirling waters serve well for this.

Are there any questions for clarification or expansion of same?

QUESTIONS & ANSWERS BY JOHN THE DIVINE

1. Where and when did breathwork originate?

Historically as a system associated with connected breath, dating back to the time period of Lemuria, a continent located in the Pacific; then passing to the civilization of Atlantis and practiced in its yogic form primarily in India; and with the Aztecs and Native Americans as an extension of the Lemurian practice and activities. Breathwork in its present form extends from Leonard Orr, the individual who rediscovered these principles in last point in time as a Native American seeking to re-create that context. First he discovered the technique of cleansing the aura through the waters, then that it was the technique of connected breath itself, then popularized it with the term *rebirthing*.

2. Would you speak about the inner breath, that point reached in breathwork where it seems that the breath is breathing us?

Physiologically, this is wherein the lungs, having fully oxygenated the physical system to capacity, reach the point of actual tissue regeneration. The breath, having penetrated dormant faculties of the circulatory system, activates the endocrine system so as to begin to purge and bring forth the natural state of regeneration and rejuvenation of the entire endocrine system, which within certain individuals lies entirely dormant. You will find that the endocrine system is not so much a usage of immunization, but more so that it works with the digestive tract, taking into the individual specific nutrient values to create the biological personality along specifically spiritual lines, thus allowing the spiritual to integrate with the physical in greater capacity. It is with the activation of the endocrine system through oxygenation, increased circulation, and increased neurological stimulation due to the relaxed state of the conscious self that the breath may achieve an autonomic state closer to the natural physiological needs of the body.* This relieves the usual stress of the conscious mind governing the muscular tissues of the diaphragm.

The experience of the inner breath is triggered on the physical level first with complete oxygenation of the system, which brings about the stimulation and greater capillary action even to the impenetrable levels of the ductless gland system itself. When these gland systems are restimulated, the response is as follows:

When the conscious self begins to enter a relaxed state, retreating more into the subconscious faculties, there is then the activation of the right-brain activities, which extend along the autonomic or parasympathetic nervous system. The autonomic system then has a more concentrated neurological activity, which is otherwise generally found in the body stored as tensions along the spine between the medulla oblongata and the coccyx.

When this tension is released, not as stress but as stimulating energy through the autonomic nervous system, then the endocrine system, which is the seat of the soul itself, can bring about the proper balance electromagnetically between all the systems, including the neurological forces and the life-force itself, which travels along the meridian systems, and the biological personality which modern science has associated with the endocrine system. And thus connected breath and other forms of kundalini breathing activate not only the glandular forces of the body physical, but through the chakras, which are the body's connection with the intangible forces of the soul, activate and integrate the body as an energy system rather than simply a chemical process.

*by shifting the autonomic nervous system from the sympathetic side ("fight or flight") to the
   parasympathetic side ("rest, digest and heal")

This is indeed as rejuvenation itself, culminating in a state of inspiration and conscious retention of all activities, since during the process the conscious mind is held in active suspension between the biological personality of the body physical and the qualities of the superconscious self.

3. **Which specific diseases of the body is breathwork best suited for?**

The most immediate results would be in the areas of cardiovascular disease, high blood pressure, or hypertension; and most diseases that are associated with stress, such as ulcerations of the abdominal walls and the closing off of any of the circulatory forces. From the altered state in breathwork, there can be the alleviation of stress as a functioning factor attributing to many degenerative diseases, such as those of cancerous and also pre-cancerous states.

Particularly in females in association with the chemical DES,[1] there can be the complete restoration of fertility and balancing of the menstrual closings. There can be the alleviation of incontinency in males and a restoration of fertility in both males and females due to increased oxygenation.

Eventually, breathwork could be applied as a healing agent for many diseases, those mentioned being the most specific diseases alleviated most immediately by any practitioner of the technique knowledgeable and skillful in the anatomy of the disease state itself.

4. **Would you comment about the use of breathwork with pregnant mothers and with children?**

There is wisdom in applying breathwork as a tool for the alleviation of tension within the first and second months of pregnancy. After that time period, the alleviation of stresses may be unwise to pursue unless in the hands of a skilled individual, since the release of tensions could have overshadowings on the embryo from the rechanneling of the mother's neurological and circulatory functions to her own needs. As postnatal care of the mother, breathwork may be immediately continued.

As to the breathwork of children, this can be applied not so much as in rhythmatics but as in a meditation, and then more so after the seventh year, as this is the critical point in the formulation of the personality. This is not to say that breathwork cannot be used for children of younger ages, but again, only in the hands of a skilled individual.

5. **How about the use of breathwork during the actual labor and birth of the child?**

The breath could be used in this context as the stimulation of the body's own natural morphines through concentration on the brow chakra and the pituitaries in same. This, then, in its own right, as rhythmatics could trigger an altered state where there is an alleviation of pain conditions.

In this context, breathwork may also be helpful in obtaining a return to the womb for the sympathetic identification with the child and with the birthing process by triggering the memory of one's own birth and bringing about the desired connection with smooth birth as an infant within self. And again, this is best only after training and in the hands of an individual skilled in these areas.

6. **Are there any instances where breathwork would be dangerous or inappropriate other than, as you mentioned, after the second month of pregnancy?**

This would vary with each individual and is of too broad a range to address here lightly. But you would find that a graduation into the process of rhythmatic breath to a level natural for the individual, so as to trigger pleasant states and pleasant attractions for breathwork, could indeed advance the individual into acceptance of deeper and deeper states of the technique. Using this graduated method of approach, again, in the hands of a skilled individual, has wisdom. There are no specific diseases that are aggravated by breathwork unless, of course, there is associated lung damage as with asthma and various other disorders.

7. **Could you say something about breathwork and the condition of asthma?**

Graduated rhythmatics, pure oxygen environments such as with the use of negative ion generators, and the taking into the system approximately three hours before breathwork of four to eight tablespoons of liquid chlorophyll with eight ounces of purified water.[2] It would indeed be well to include this program in all breathwork sessions, for you will find that chlorophyll is but one molecular structure removed from hemoglobin, or blood itself.* Chlorophyll, which may be found most suitably in the juice of wheatgrass, certain algaes or spirulina, and sprouts and leafy vegetables, helps greatly to increase the oxygenation of the system.

8. **Could you elaborate about the spiritual states connected with the inner breath and the more spiritual aspects of the breath, such as in the Bible verse, "And God breathed into [man] the breath of life"?**[3]

You will find that the inner breath, when you obtain it, is both a conscious and a physiological process. The soul's force is indeed independent of any process, meditation, or element of prayer, for the soul itself as the Divine Self is an energy unto itself with which you integrate and which you all indeed are seeking to become. Breathwork and the use of the chakras mentioned are but as activities for the isolation of levels of that consciousness to where they integrate within the currently functioning conscious self so that ye may become more and more the servant of God. And God is love.

The breath of life as was breathed into Adam in those days was more so that he could become a living soul. This does not speak of the physical breath in association to the oxygen and the physiological process, but more so of the inner life. That is the total integration of mind, body, and spirit and activation of the Christ Principle itself within ye, becoming knowledgeable of thine own aspect of God, who indeed is love. And love is harmony.

---

*Hemoglobin is the iron-containing protein in red blood cells. It transports oxygen from the lungs to the rest of the body, such as to the muscles, where it releases the oxygen load.

The inner breath is described as but the harmonics between the physiological personality, the conscious self, and then indeed the activities of the soul—harmony between these three forces of body, mind, and spirit. Therefore this becomes the practical love of self, "Love thy neighbor as thyself."[4]

This is not a selfishness, the desire only of physical survival, but it is the desire to promote health and healing through understanding that ye may be of greater capacity in service unto others. As ye increase thine own vitality, this can be of the purpose so as to be more vital and more of an inspiration to others of the harmony that is God.

10. Could you speak of the possibility of individuals, through the processes of connected breathing and rejuvenation, attaining the state of biological immortality?

Biological immortality is actually little more than the constant regeneration of the physical form as well as obeying the laws of God. Rhythmatic breathing, therefore, enhances the context of the proper dietary mode, which, according to the law of God, "Thou shalt not kill," would be more along the lines of the vegetarian diet.

[At this point, the discourse was interrupted by the spirit Tom McPherson.]

❧—❦ ❧—❦ ❧—❦

TOM McPHERSON
On Life Extension with Questions & Answers

Greetings! McPherson here.

How are the lot of you doing out there? I didn't mean to interrupt John's discourse, but I wish to come through to relay a bit of information in relation to biological immortality.

First of all, for those of you who don't know me, my name is Tom McPherson. I'm a spirit and, being on this side, I believe you can relate to the fact that I didn't make biological immortality. But anyway, that was my problem and not yours—you still have a fighting chance for it, shall we say.

Biological immortality, as John was saying, is little more than continuous tissue regeneration, which is accomplishable, for instance, in the growing of limbs on frogs, and so on. Recently you've been able to do this with mammals through the stimulation of electricity by planting electrodes and then directing low-voltage electricity along the neurological tissues. This is correctly based upon the theory that the blood plasma is the source of a nonstructured DNA molecule that contains all of the cellular memory necessary for the duplication of tissues. Whether it be bone marrow or heart tissues, the building blocks are contained therein.

Now then, the key to life extension, as John began to point out, lies in the obeying of God's laws. And if you obey the law that thou shalt not kill, then you would lean more toward the vegetarian diet and that chlorophyll is only one atom removed from the molecular structure of blood. And so for all you "green vampires" out there, your concentration on the vegetarian diet for gaining a higher enzyme content closer in substance to the blood plasma makes for the easier translation into cell and tissue regeneration.

Then, too, your breathwork alleviates the tension that ages the physical body and causes blockages in the neurological tissues. Breathwork also produces complete circulation for the activation of the enzyme system for improved digestion of foodstuffs. It does this by reactivating the proper functioning of the endocrine system, which is digestive and not immunitive,* so that actually the stomach should be little more than a tube through which liquids pass. The ideal diet is basically liquified protein from seed sources, broken down through processes of fermentation so as to become yogurt-like, and liquids with lots of chlorophyll and juices. So you would continue to take protein from non-meat sources and sugars from fruit sources to produce the context of longevity to 125 or 150 years.

You will notice the vegetarian takes on the leaner look. The stomach is only expanded and swelled out when you start stuffing yourself with meats, producing the sag about the midsection which is associated with age and poor posture, and so on.

1. What might be the appropriate content of a lifestyle that approaches forever? What would we do with our time here on this planet? Is there that much work to be done?

In order to completely get all the work done? All of you would have to live about five thousand years to burn off the karmic implications there! The British are still around, so about another ten-thousand there[1]...

Yes, there are plenty of things to do. Just mastering this plane is quite involved, to be frank. As to life extension on this plane, actually what would transpire is that this would take you on into the soul's forces. You would start mastering a whole new host of sensitivities. For instance, once you got the physical body aligned and attuned, all of its chakric centers together, the soul's forces would start pouring in, so to say, and you would start having prognostic dreams, and so on.

Prognostic dreams, by the way, are little more than one of the soul's senses. For instance, when you fly an airplane, do you not need radar for flying at speeds that the

*The endocrine system regulates digestive function by secreting hormones. It also provides the key communication and control link between the nervous system and bodily functions such as reproduction, immunity, metabolism, and behavior.

body is not used to? Therefore, when you start soul-traveling around, which is obtainable, mind you, you need an extra sense, an ESP*, to be able to travel at those faster-than-light speeds. So ESP is little more than your sensory radar for when your physical body is able to teleport around, so to say, and levitate, etc. So yes, unless you think you can master levitation in ten easy lessons, life extension has its practicalities.

2. How is levitation associated with life extension?

Easy. Once the body is attuned to the capacity of life extension, you need a quick way to get around, so to say, to accomplish certain acts. Levitation is merely a byproduct of aligning the physical body with the higher energies. For instance, there is a constant flow of electricity that passes through your body and through the atmosphere at all times. Once the body is aligned and adapted to the new metabolism, you can actually tune into those energies to attain levitation.

3. Can you use levitation as a process for attaining life extension?

To a degree, yes, as you would find in the following manner. (How shall I put this?) You use the inner ear for balance and for walking with gravity, do you not? Is that not the physiological form of balancing the self in gravity? The physically immortalized body can levitate itself from gravity by channeling circulatory flow to specific portions of the endocrine system to balance itself the same way as when you use your inner ear to curve-form your body to balance yourself in gravity so you don't fall flat on your face. We use the endocrine system and the seven chakras to obtain balance while in levitation. Also, of course, the physically immortalized body has complete mastery of the blood flow—you might call it your hydraulic system for balancing yourself in gravity.

4. Do you feel there are certain vitamins, like the megavitamin therapy that's so popular, that can support life extension?

I think life extension comes through the mastery of your physical body and the

---

*Extra-sensory perception

return to a more natural and better diet. Megavitamin therapy is a system for replenishing depletions and reopening the body to its full capacity. It's a sort of reminder that your body needs those vitamins since it is so atrophied. Your bodies will basically rob themselves of energy from different sources to stay alive, like robbing Peter to pay Paul, which is the aging process.

5. Do you feel that we will keep going through reincarnation until we master the physical body?

No, it's not necessary to obtain physical mastery to gain spiritual mastery. It's the path of some people, so to say. Biological immortality is merely an expression of totally anchoring the soul on this plane. Jesus did it. So can you. If you live well and long, you may fulfill your karma and indeed transcend this plane. You may also choose the option of being able to astral-project and then not checking back in!

In any case, what you need to do is to align yourself, to be at peace with your physical form and at peace with your spiritual existence, so that when the time of physical passing comes, be it stepping out in front of a truck, dying of pneumonia, or being a little old gray-haired lady who leaves in her sleep, you have no fear of physical passing. You shouldn't think in terms of conscious choice, as in, "Oh, I want to exit the physical plane on the thirtieth of January in 1984," so to say. It's leaving with consciousness rather than consciously picking a date.

6. What is it that you can do over here that you can't do on that side? What's the reason for incarnating?

You have a broader choice of activity. If you're a saint on this side, all you can be is "good, gooder or goodest!" Having a physical body is actually an advantage.

What we have over here that you also have is a personality, which is an advantage and a disadvantage. It allows me to speak and communicate, to have an ego and to not have an ego at the same time. You all have a physical body. You can travel around on the earth plane, experience pain and hunger. You can experience traveling from a Stone Age culture to the most advanced technology on the planet. The advantages of having a physical form are in the ability to function on the material plane and in dealing with karma.

The key thing is that almost anything in the spiritual realms can indeed be experienced from the vantage of the physical plane. You see, the advantage is that you have a point of emphasis, you have a conscious choice of limitation or lack thereof. In other words, you actually have privacy to a degree. And you have choice of tuning in or tuning out, a rather unique spectrum of free will, so to say. However, you also have the capacity of astral projection into higher realms, so while still being physically incarnate you can experience all the beauty of the spiritual realms.

7. **About karma, you say it's easier to work out karma while being a physical being. What about a nonphysical being? How easy is it to work out whatever karma you still have?**

Bloody well difficult! Because, you see, what we are dependent on for the burning off of karma in the discarnate state is the experience of the individuals to whom we give guidance. And as you stumble along over there, we bite our nails many a day!

For clarity, though, it's that we over here possess no physical body, only a personality. And the personality is within the context of karma itself. It is actually the mold or shape that karma takes.

You, however, have a physical body, you have a brand new personality, you have an instrument for burning off karma, while we must more or less stand on the sidelines and observe your progress or regression without direct intercession. It's the equivalent of the only thing you can do at a football game, which is to shout and scream in an attempt to stimulate the team, but you cannot make the plays yourself. Noninterference to a degree is mandatory unless it is within the limits of your conscious permission.

8. **Why haven't you chosen to incarnate, then, if it seems like the better way?**

Because I'm an Irishman and for the past forty years the British Empire has been all over the planet and I haven't found a decent place to incarnate![1] That's part of the reason. But the actual reason is that I experienced a very ribald lifetime in Atlantis but it was a very drab lifetime—I developed absolutely no humor. And so therefore in the personality I currently occupy as Tom McPherson, I've developed quite a humor, so to say, or I like to think of myself that way.

But I still need a backdrop similar to Atlantis in terms of a higher degree of technology and society similar to Atlantis to fulfill the rest of my karma, and you haven't developed that yet. In other words, you are bloody well preparing the way for my own reincarnation with the various advancements you are making. So get busy, you inventors. I'm cheering you on over here. The ball is in your court!

9. **Can breathwork be considered the only technique necessary to work out all the karma we have so that we won't have to reincarnate on this plane?**

No, not at all. There is no one particular technique that alleviates all your karma except basically the law of grace. Breathwork is basically a tune-up for the personality, so to speak, so that it works well with the law of grace. It can give you health and vitality. It can give you more to share of yourself. It helps you develop an altruistic nature.

But it's not the only tool that you would need to fulfill your karma, so to say, although it is an excellent tool to bring you closer to it. Certainly the practice of meditation, the art of self-giving (karma yoga), and the other yogic arts which come to us from the East are excellent tools. Life is probably the only tool. The law of grace is basically the ability to forgive and forget other individuals, to work with the higher tools of patience, wisdom, and service to others, and above all, to develop a loving nature.

I believe I have to be going now. It's been very pleasant speaking to the lot of you. I wish you all a good day!

JOHN THE DIVINE
Closing

Hail! You will find that even as ye are of one mind yet with many thoughts, so in turn there is but one God with many souls, so that each of you is as a thought within the Mind of God.

Even as thoughts may become synthesized so as to create a new thought independent of the original two, so in turn does each one of you merge to become that particular focus which is God in thy Higher Self. And each must manifest that nature upon this plane so as to spiritualize both the personality and the environment that you inhabit, creating an environment of light and love.

For indeed, God is love, love is harmony, and harmony begets peace.

God bless you. Amen.

❧—❧ ❧—❧ ❧—❧

THE ESSENE REBIRTH
THROUGH MICHAEL RICHARD

BY
KATHERINE THE HEALER

AND
JOHN THE BAPTIST

❧—❧ ❧—❧ ❧—❧

SAN DIEGO, CALIFORNIA
MARCH 1, 1981

❧—❧ ❧—❧ ❧—❧

EDITOR'S NOTE: On March 1, 1981, north of San Diego, California, under the full moon, twenty-one people gathered to learn about and to practice healing through breath, sound and water as performed by the Essenes over two thousand years ago. One week earlier, John the Baptist through Michael Richard had suggested this meeting as an opportune time for teachings to come through. These teachings were to elaborate on the practices referred to in the previously released discourses. First we were instructed by one known as Katherine the Healer through Michael to set ourselves up with seven of us supporting Michael in the warm water of a hot tub, while we all began a flowing connected breath. We were instructed to align ourselves for the sending of energy through Michael and we used the chanting of the AUM to unify our energy.[1] Michael then delivered the teaching from John the Baptist.

KATHERINE THE HEALER
Essene Rebirth & Breathwork Guidelines

Placing of the Hands

The one at the head supports the head alone. The two at the shoulders (one on each side) place one hand behind the nape of the neck and one hand at the shoulder. It is not necessary to raise the body out of the water or to support it physically. The support should be by way of light touch. The support comes from within and from the heart. Next, two support the middle, with one hand at the place corresponding to the kidneys and the other hand supporting the buttocks. The third individual on each side is to support the upper thigh with one hand and the knee with the other.

Cleansing of the Breath

Among those in the tub at this time, there needs to be a cleansing of the breath. This can be performed by taking three deep breaths in unison. This will serve to cleanse the breath. At the same time, there must be unity of thought and purpose. With the exhale, release all blockages, both mental and physical. Before taking the three breaths, intuitively scan your bodies. Do that at this time. Any dim or gray areas that you intuitively feel as you mentally scan up and down your bodies are areas of energy blockage. Direct your energy to those areas, pull them up and release them with your breath. When each individual has completed the scan, unify your breathing for the three breaths. Follow the one at the head.

Aligning of the Breathworker

This cleansing and purification is necessary on the part of all those who would become breathworkers. It is necessary that the breathworker align their own being first. This is the procedure. This scanning procedure can be followed both during wet and dry breathwork sessions. First, there is an invocation of light and energy for the purification of the room (when done dry) and of the water (when wet), followed by an inner search and intuitive cleansing of the body by the breathworker to remove blockages. This can be accomplished as the participant begins a very slow process of the breath. It is essential that the breathworkers be aware of their own process and their own presence in the breathwork. Centeredness and clarity are required at all times.

Physical clarity is necessary so that the physical being of the breathworker—any aches and pains or other physical disturbances—do not enter into the process any more than is necessary to maintain comfort of the breathworker. Breathwork should not be used if either the breathworker or the participant is not comfortable and clear.

It is respectful, and it is the greatest service the breathworker can render, to state in advance any lack of clarity, lack of centeredness. If the breathwork process is not cleared by verbal command, the session should not proceed. It is the responsibility of the breathworker to ensure clarity. All other considerations must be secondary.

Passing of the Hands

Often preceding the breathwork, it is beneficial to have the client or the friend breathe through their own body. And as they initially begin breathing, they may be given verbal commands. Commands to search their body for areas of blockage are given and then energy is guided into these areas. A similar technique may be used for the scanning of the finer mental and emotional bodies. During this time the breathworker may also, once clear, move the hands lightly up the body in such a way as to intuitively feel blockages in the body.

Release of those blockages can be attained by moving from the feet toward the head, releasing the energy through the crown chakra while balancing the right hand to the left side of the body and the left hand to the right side of the body and moving upward. The points that will be necessary for concentration of this light touch procedure will be apparent to the breathworker if the breathworker is clear. Follow your intuition. Moving up the body, touch those points which you intuitively feel need to be touched. Pressure is not necessary but may be appropriate in some circumstances.

Intuition

Again, the service that you do is intuitive. Release yourself to channel the healing energy of God's Source in all that comes through you. Release yourselves from ego-centeredness and from connection to your own process. As you work, you are an instrument of the Creative Mind and of the intuitive creative force of the universe, which is known as thought, which is known as Godhead, which is known as the inner voice. Follow it. Its guidance is true and clear. That is why it is essential for you to clear yourselves first in order for the intuitive channels and the healing light to flow clearly and concisely through you without your own internal blockages.

Remember always during the process that all is thought. All that is necessary for thought to be realized in physical manifestation is verbalization. The word is what *is*; thus the verbal clearing of the room or the water before the rebirth. If the facilitator does not feel clear, their own clearing process must be undertaken first so that they may correctly and intuitively read the room for its innate feeling vibration.

Intentions of the Breathwork Session

Often before the session begins, it may be necessary for the breathworker to discuss what the goals are and learn what the participant intends to take place during the session. This is often a way of avoiding unnecessary drama, which we have all experienced. To set forth a plan of action and specific goals will do two things. It will enable the participant to design a breathwork according to their greatest need at that moment. It will also enable the participant to gain greater relaxation so that they feel they have some control over the direction of the session. Again, thought is creative. One thing may be expressed verbally and quite another may come out in the session. The breathworker must know that the message was received on the level of thought even if it was "stuffed" on the level of verbalization.

Therefore, the breathworker should not attempt to control the direction of the session once the process has begun, but should serve from time to time to guide the person in the direction of the stated purpose of the session. One method of accomplishing this is by asking certain questions. For instance, if the person wants to work on the level of letting go of irrational fear, then the breathworker might work intuitively by bringing up points dealing with fear, with separation, with frustration—the things that build fear. If by common agreement you are dealing with a physical problem, the breathworker might guide the participant's attention and breathing to those areas of the body indicated by the stated intention.

This vocalization will produce many beneficial results. It will also add credence to the definite sequence of events as they unfold during the process. Many who are not now accepting the process do so for its seeming open-endedness. The process in and of itself is an open-ended one for spiritual awakening, physical mastery, emotional clearing, and psychic attunement. However, it can and should be used on the level of specific goals in all of these areas.

Sealing the Session

When it has been determined by both parties that the energy of the session has subsided and the various releasing cycles have reached their completion, it is then both wise and beneficial to do a sealing procedure. This may be done in the following manner:

As the breathworker, you place your right hand at the coccyx or, if more convenient, at the pelvic bone just below the navel of the participant. Place your left hand very lightly at the third-eye point or at the top of the spine at the medulla. Hold these positions for a few moments and breathe, allowing the balancing energy to flow through you. Direct the person toward grounding and returning fully to their presence in the body.

Suggest to them that they are complete, that they are firmly anchored on Mother Earth, that their aura is now sealed. Also suggest that they will retain all the benefits and memory of their experience. This effectively seals the session. This or other sealing and completing techniques should be applied after every session.

Support of the Body in the Water

Support should be equal on both sides, left and right. Follow your own intuitive guidelines as to the amount of support necessary. Be attuned most directly with that individual across from you. Adjust your levels of support, each of you, up and down until you know that you are supporting equally on both sides. Adjust the levels of support according to intuition by watching the third eye of that individual opposite. [Those supporting Michael adjust their levels of support.] Perfect. That is fine. Now that your intuitive senses are functioning perfectly, follow them completely.

To avoid tensions building up in the body, feel free to adjust your bodies while releasing your support with your physical hands. Do not remove your support on the spiritual and psychic levels. Stay connected and you can feel free to move the physical body as necessary. After all, you are essentially spirit; the body functions at your needs. If it is uncomfortable, go within yourselves and search for the uncomfortability. It is possible to release all feelings of stress within the body arising from your support by going within yourself and looking at your willingness to support on a spiritual, psychic, and physical level. Plant that particle, remove that energy blockage and you will feel greater relaxation and comfort in your position of support.

❖──❖ ❖──❖ ❖──❖
·

THE ESSENE REBIRTH

At this time I'd like you to do some chanting, achieving a greater sense of unity through the voice. Also at this time, I wish you to dispel all existing doubts, and I ask only that all of those present increase their level of faith. [All present chant:]

"AAAUUUMMMMMM"

When you AUM, send the vibration through the heart into Michael.

"AAAUUUMMMMMM"

Continue to focus on the third eye of each other.

"AAAUUUMMMMMM"

There is a greeting that comes to all who are present. I know of your love and I know of your hearts. Greetings to all of you. Your faith is great. And your initiations are complete, all of you, through your expression of faith here tonight.

We will now chant seven AUMs focusing on the seven chakras, starting with the base chakra, following my lead. The sound will be incremented upward each time and we will use the visualization of the light ray corresponding to each chakra. Go within your chest; the sound will come from the heart chakra. Open your throat; let it flow out naturally and easily.

You are all angels with perfect voices. Allow your divinity to be expressed through sound. Come from deep within your own heart center.

Vibrate the tones down until you feel your heart vibrate. Then move the sounds down until you feel the kundalini chakra at the base of the spine begin to vibrate. Visualize a white light emanating from that center.

"AAAUUUMMMMMMM"

Now vibrate the sound at the sexual chakra and imagine an emanation of the violet color from that center.

"AAAUUUMMMMMMM"

Raise the vibration to the center of life-force at the solar plexus. The colors are purple with gold. The sound is in your heart. Feel the vibration in that center.

"AAAUUUMMMMMMM"

Move the vibration up to the heart chakra. The glow of light there is a rose pink. Feel the vibration in your heart; hear it in your heart. The sounds may not sound always alike. Attune to the vibrations of those around you first. Your own sounds will vibrate in unison regardless of your ear tone. Follow the vibration of your own heart. As each of you possesses an individual vibration, so each of you individually manifests God through your God centers.*

"AAAUUUMMMMMMM"

Now move the sound up into the throat chakra or to the area corresponding to the mouth, nose, and throat. Do not emphasize the throat; emphasize the heart. Let the vibration flow from the heart into the vocal cords. Visualize a rich blue color at this chakra.

"AAAUUUMMMMMMM"

Now bring the energy up to the third eye. The light emanation is emerald green. Feel the energy coming up from your heart, flowing up your spine, flowing into your third eye, creating sound that is infinite.

*chakras

"AAAUUUMMMMMM"

And finally, release your voice to the golden yellow sun of the crown chakra. You are all angels. It shows in your voices. You are beginning to feel your presence now and with one another before.

Open your heart, open yourselves completely. Feel with one another. All are one. All is vibrational energy. Those who join the vibration, the sound of Universal Consciousness, join the God that they manifest along with all other manifestations on the planet.

This will necessarily be a very high pitch, to be held only for a few moments, only for one breath. Unify yourselves completely. You are very close now. You are all one. Feel the vibration.

"AAAUUUMMMMMM"

When doing breathwork and supporting Godhead in this fashion, you will move in unison from the base-of-the-spine chakra to the crown chakra, utilizing these modulated sounds and color visualizations. Again, the vibration is of primary importance, not what your ear hears. Sense the vibration with your etheric being. The vibration of your own voice will follow.[1]

❖—❖ ❖—❖ ❖—❖

JOHN THE BAPTIST
Teaching the Light

In order that you follow God, in order that you be children and teachers of the Way, of the Light, you must have faith in yourselves. There is no one who can guide you, there is no one who can give you anything. You are not going anywhere. You are beings of light in total perfection at this moment and at every moment. All that you have ever been, all that you ever will be, is now.

What becomes necessary for you to follow the Light is that you release yourselves from the drama, from all that does not serve you, be it physical, mental, or psychic. The time has come for each of you to accept not me, not Michael, not Cochise, not Yogananda,[1] not Jesus, not Sivananda[2]—if you accept us as other than yourselves. We are your guides.

Your guides assist you and walk by your sides. They do not walk in front of you, nor do they drag you bodily. The time for you to release yourselves is now. The games with which you choose to engulf yourselves are what is known in all religions, in all faiths, as hell. The hell is within you, as is bliss, as is Nirvana, as is heaven. The time for you to get it is now.

Many times we have come together as disciples, as students, as friends, as teachers. Most often, the role most comfortable for all of us has been that of student, that of learner. The time is now for each of you to know that you are complete, to have faith in your own abilities to guide yourselves.

Along the path, many of you have served as teachers. Some of you at this time are becoming aware of the teachers that you yourselves were in past lifetimes. Others of you will become aware of the teachers you will be in what is called future time.

You will experience states of past and future time until you accept that you are the teachers at whose feet you so quickly prostrate yourselves. Prostration is a sign of love.

It is a sign of servitude. When you bow, bow to your own Inner Christ, bow to your Self. You are all that is. When that realization comes, then you will truly know all there is to know. All there is to know is now. All masters are you.

From time to time, all of you will receive guidance that you must communicate from your heart to others, understanding fully that what comes, comes from God through you as a manifestation of God. There is no separation between the two. If separation exists within your own minds, there will be no now for you. You are now. If others come to you, you are the ones who can teach. The teacher is the greatest student of them all. The teacher uses each of you. The teacher within is not teaching another, but is in fact teaching you. You teach through allowing the channel to open through you, through being, realizing in your own heart in faith deep within your beings the oneness of you, the oneness of I AM, the oneness of "all who come through the Father, come through me."[3]

You will fully become the student. Teach as the student. Follow your inner guides; they will teach you first. You are merely a channel, if you must believe of yourself that way. You are all that you can be, now. Get that. Now is all there is!

Be the student forever. Teach, each of you, what you can and what you are certain of. You are fully manifested and have all knowledge now. You have knowledge of yourselves as light beings, knowledge of each other as complete and whole. What you see before you is always natural. What is, is always Godhead. Always, all that is before you is to present you, the student, with the tools to spread the Word.

Always remember that you are complete whether you practice your trade, your profession, whether you do nothing. The mode that you have chosen is holy, is appropriate, is where the greatest manifestation of Godhead will exist and will be realized. Therefore, as you exist in the world, please acknowledge Godhead, acknowledge that where you are at this moment is all that you can be. You are perfect. Do not cloister yourselves. Do not seclude yourselves.

There is in the New Age no room for the elitism that destroyed civilizations that have come before and attempted to express God-realization on the physical plane.

At the point at which hierarchy was established within the Lemurian, Atlantean, Roman, Grecian, Egyptian, Mayan, all of what are called primitive cultures, elitism began the destruction of full realization of Godhead. That is the symbolic falling out of the Garden of Eden in the New Age. Understand that.

You are all Godhead. Those who are to follow are equal and are high manifestations of Godhead. The task before you is to lead from spiritual enlightenment. Enlightenment means, "I serve God through serving myself, my own higher goals," and by allowing full manifestation of Godhead from all those in your lives.

All that is, is ultimately good. All that is, is ultimately a manifestation of Christ Consciousness. All is one. Express not your own inner judgments, your own inner peevishness. Come forth as children of God. Allow yourselves to express what you feel as human beings, but recognize that all expressions through you, as all expressions through every other human being, when they seem to be blocking your progress, are actually advancing it.

All beings of light must shine forth in the darkness. Bring forth within yourselves the light deep within you that will allow you to bring out your Christ Consciousness. As it flows, accept what is within yourself. All that you express—whether on the physical, whether verbally, whether mentally, in terms of control, in terms of unloving attitudes, in terms of physical abuse of yourselves and others—is the cleansing that you, as spiritual beings working toward greater and greater pure knowledge of Godhead, are getting rid of.

Do not deny within yourself those things that you would like most to be rid of. Denial will continue to keep them buried within you and will allow you to experience the pain and frustration, the hell that you are holding inside. Release those emotions, have faith in yourself, turn to your own inner being.

Come forth with all that you are now, but do not deny those things that come also as an expression of your Godhead. Those who achieve physical, mental, and spiritual mastery will ascend to the throne to sit by the side of all masters. Self-expression is the way. The key to self-expression is to remember at all times that you are expressing God within. Release your greatest fears.

Release is not a mental process. Release is not lying on the ground prostrated in front of someone to give your life to them. You must give light to yourself! You are Christ Consciousness. Full realization of that will come within this lifetime for each of you if you keep your mind's eye centered on Christ Consciousness and on the full realization that each of you is a manifestation of Godhead. Do not deny yourselves. Do not deny yourselves!

Only know that as you teach, so you learn. As you express, you will learn more about yourselves, about the Christ that dwells within. As you allow free expression around you by those you love and care for, without judgment, without qualification, and unconditionally, you will find within yourself the student of Christ Consciousness.

Go within yourselves. Support each other. The work that you do at this time— be it in an office, be it driving a truck, be it doing the dishes, anything you do—is God-manifestation. Be with it. Know that though you may feel uncomfortable at certain times where you are, you are being guided to be there. Do not look to those around you to judge what you do, who you are, what you feel, or what you can be. You are where you are because you will learn the most from that situation. You will learn from that situation all that is necessary before you are released from that situation. If not, that situation will again arise for you.

One tool that you all have at your disposal now is to look at the patterning of your lives. You are constructing them with your own higher thought-being. If you find you are repeating, you must look for the lesson, not the escape route. For there is only one escape route, and it is an escape into light. It is an escape that is an awakening of higher levels of consciousness and awareness. If you have chosen for yourselves a path a second time around or a third time around, know that you must go within, that as soon as you have accepted what you are most attempting to learn, you will be released from that path. This is true in terms of worldly work, in terms of relationships, in terms of money, in terms of all that is. Once those higher realizations have been expressed and those lower feelings and emotions and blockages have been released, you will experience heaven.

When all that you feel is oneness with all that is, and you have fully accepted that you are the Christ that cometh, you will begin to walk the gilded path of the masters. And many such will come before you. Many of you will be chosen to go before the masses as Buddha did, as Lord Krishna did, as Yogananda did, as Jesus did, as all the great earthly masters have done.

This is a time of greater and greater God-realization, a time of miracles. You are the vehicles. You have willingly chosen to be here in faith. You have chosen to come together to support each and every one of you in completeness and God-manifestation. Remind each other of your purposes. Accept about each other that you are complete at every moment and perfect beings at every moment. Do not feel yourself nor your friends nor anyone you meet to be incomplete, to be ill in any way. With this in mind, each of you will become a healer. For the healing process only requires that you believe in the wholeness, the perfection of all that is right now. Remove the laws of imperfection that bind you, that bind others, and you have achieved Christ Consciousness.

Do not accept any other view but that which you know to be true. Go within yourselves. Do not deny the Christ within you. Each time you allow yourselves to destroy what you build due to fear, due to insecurity, due to a sense of lack, you sin against Christ in the sense that you sin against yourself. There is no God outside of you. Look within. Do not deny yourselves. Each of you is a child of light. Each of you possesses the Spirit. Express this as individuals and express it through your community. Do what you do with heart, with certainty, and with the knowledge that you are Christ Consciousness.

All that is, is within you now. Tonight we are here to symbolically free ourselves from self-imposed bondage. There is none here who can release you but yourselves. There is none here who can accept your purity but you. All here are here, and by their presence have agreed, to support one another in God-realization. Know that they are with you. Feel it within yourselves.

The baptism of water is symbolic of full acceptance of yourselves as Christ Consciousness manifested on this plane. Each of you has work to do. Express yourselves individually and as a community. Support one another in your journeys. Work each day.

Tell yourselves—deep within yourselves until you know it, as you really do know—that you are Sons and Daughters of God, that you are Christ manifest. Each of you is a being of light. Be with it, be one with it. It is your True Self.

Each of you flows deep within my heart. I flow deep within yours. Be as you are: Christ Consciousness at this moment.

The more that you realize and express, the more that you will realize miracles in your lifetime, miracles of a very ordinary quality. God will work because you will work.

Your work shall not be judged by its title nor its sum. Your work will be judged by you. You stand in final judgment of yourself. You will be in physical, mental, and spiritual hell until you release all judgments upon yourself that see you as anything less than Christ manifest.

Look not in your own hell. That is all the hell there is. Lift your spirits. Go through the lessons, the teachings, and the everyday life of a master. All of you are such.

Go forth in peace and in certainty. And you need never walk alone, for we are with you. Amen.

❧—❧ ❧—❧ ❧—❧

CHAPTER 1

Preface ~ 2006

1. See Sondra Ray's book, *Loving Relationships*.

2. For more on Kevin Ryerson, visit www.KevinRyerson.com.

3. For more on the Essenes and to read *The Essene Gospels of Peace*, visit www.TheNazareneWay.com.

4. For more on Dr. Andrew Weil, visit www.DrWeilSelfHealing.com. Listen to his CD album, *Breathing: The Masterkey to Self Healing*.

5. Visit Michael Grant White's extensive optimal breathing development web site at www.Breathing.com.

6. Breathwork modalities: Visit Dan Brulé's www.BreathMastery.com; the Holotropic Breathwork of Dr. Stanislav Grof at www.Breathwork.com; Leonard Orr's rebirthing site, www.LeonardOrr.com. and my site: www.IntegralBreathwork.com.

CHAPTER 2

Introduction ~ 1982

1. Akashic Records. (*Akasha* is a Sanskrit word meaning "sky," "space" or "ether.") References to these etheric records exist in all cultures. The belief is that each soul records every moment of their existence in what the Bible calls *The Book of Life*, and if one can attune oneself properly, one can read from that book.

CHAPTER 4

Breathwork's Ancient History

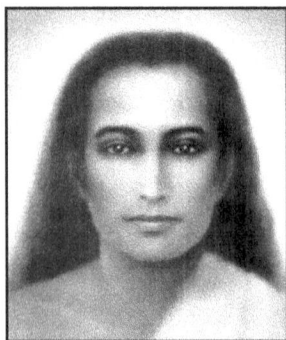

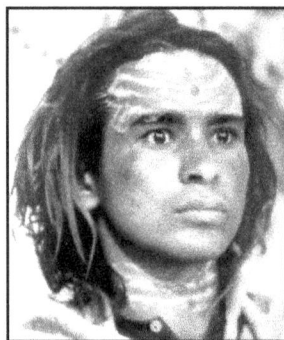

1. The revered Himalayan adept known as **Babaji** (l., c. 1860–1922) is spoken of vividly in Yogananda's *Autobiography of a Yogi*. Raj Yogi Sri Lord Haidiyakhandi Bhole Baba (Babaji) (r., 1970–1984) is this same Babaji in his last incarnation, who is said to have emerged from a Himalayan cave as a fully formed young adult. Many of the original rebirthers at that time were

devotees of this master and felt that he sponsored breathwork. Many traveled to India to have darshan with him and to chant "OM NAMAH SHIVAYA." For more extensive info, visit: www.PolaChurchill.com, or you can search the above long name on Facebook.

2. Thoth. (THŎTH, T OT), in Egyptian religion, god of wisdom and magic. A patron of learning, alchemy and the arts, he was credited with many inventions, including writing, geometry and astronomy. Thoth was also a messenger and scribe for the gods. He was identified by the Greeks and named Hermes Trismegistus (*Thrice Greatest*). See Hermetic books, especially *The Emerald Tablet*. Often represented as an ibis-headed man.

3. Rajneesh Chandra Mohan Jain (1931–1990), better known during the 1970s as Bhagwan Shree Rajneesh, and later as Osho. He was an Eastern Indian spiritual teacher, or guru. He lived in India and the United States and was the spiritual head of the Osho-Rajneesh movement, a controversial new religious movement. For a full biography, go to www.Answers.com/Rajneesh.

4. Leboyer Method. See *Birth Without Violence* by Frederick Leboyer. This book was considered "the bible" by early breathworkers.

CHAPTERS 8–9

Physiology of Breathwork & Chakra Work, Questions & Answers

1. DES: diethylstilbestrol, a colorless crystalline synthetic compound ($C_{18}H_{20}O_2$) used as a potent estrogen but contraindicated in pregnancy for its tendency to cause cancer or birth defects in offspring.

2. The recommended dosage is 4–8 tablespoons of liquid chlorophyll. If using E3Live liquid blue-green algae, use 2 or more tablespoons in water.

3. Reference to Genesis 2:7.

4. Reference to Matthew 5:43.

CHAPTER 10

On Life Extension with Questions & Answers

1. This is an attempt at humor by Tom, as he refers to the long-standing rivalry between the Irish and the British.

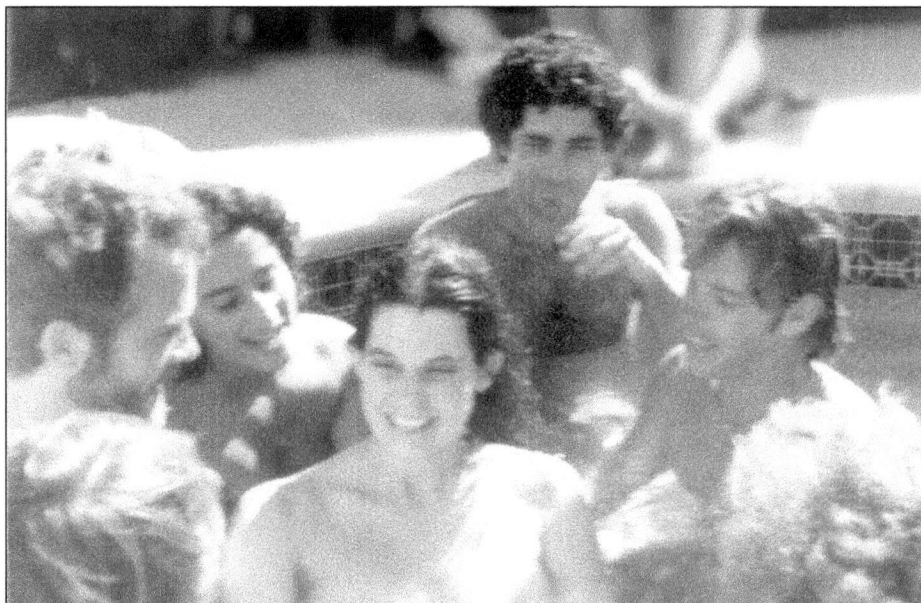

The occasion was a birthday celebration for the lady in the center. It was her request that we experience this free of clothing. While we opted to use clothing for most of these rituals, there was an innocent, Edenic consciousness among us at that time, and an open naturist attitude toward nudity.

They were naked... and were not ashamed (Genesis 2:25).
An Essene Rebirth circa 1984. *(See Note 12 below and right).*

CHAPTER 11

Essene Rebirth & Breathwork Guidelines

1. AUM also OM (O̅M) n. *Hinduism & Buddhism.* The supreme and most sacred syllable, consisting in Sanskrit of the three sounds *(ah), (oh-u),* and *(mm),* representing various fundamental triads (i.e., Father, Son, and Holy Spirit or Brahma, Vishnu, and Shiva). Believed to be the spoken essence of the universe, it is sounded as a mantra and in invocations and blessings. In the chanting portion of the Essene Rebirth, I have drawn out the phonetic spelling with the *mmmm* twice as long as the *au.* This is the extended resonating of the Omega, or Mother, aspect for the anchoring of Spirit (Alpha, Father, *ah*) into the physical.

CHAPTER 12

The Essene Rebirth

1. The above photo was taken just after an Essene Rebirth ritual done in San Diego, California. Notice the pure joy on our faces, especially the lady in the center, who has just emerged from the ceremony after we held her in the water and did the breathing and chanting as prescribed in this chapter. That's me in profile on the left. Michael Richard, the mediums who delivered the words of Katherine the Healer and John the Baptist recorded here, is with the dark hair in the upper right. Two other friends I remember are Wendy and Edward on both sides of Michael. The ceremony took about an hour.

CHAPTER 13

Teaching the Light

1. Yogananda. (Paramahansa Yogananda, 1893–1952). Eastern Indian mystic. Born in India of a Kshatriya (warrior caste) family. Before attending Calcutta University he met his guru, Sri Yukteswar. In 1917, he founded the Yogada Satsang School for boys in Calcutta. In 1920, he went to the United States, where he lectured widely, teaching a sacred technique of meditation he called *kriya yoga.* He founded the Self-Realization Fellowship to carry on his work, and lived in the U.S. until his death. His organization, which has headquarters in Los Angeles, has centers throughout the world. See his *Autobiography of a Yogi* (1946).

2. Sivananda. (Swami Sivananda Saraswati, 1887–1963). A Hindu by birth, he is a well-known proponent of yoga and vedanta. Sivananda performed austerities for many years. In 1936, he founded the Divine Life Society, a new religious movement, on the banks of the Ganges. Among his disciples were the young U.G. Krishnamurti, and Swami Satyananda Saraswati, founder of Satyananda Yoga. He wrote excellent books on Hinduism and closely followed the Adviata philosophy. Many of his books are available on the web at www.dlshq.org. On July 14, 1963, the Great Soul Swami Sivananda entered Mahasamadhi (departure of a Self-realized saint from his mortal coil).

3. Reference to John 6:44.

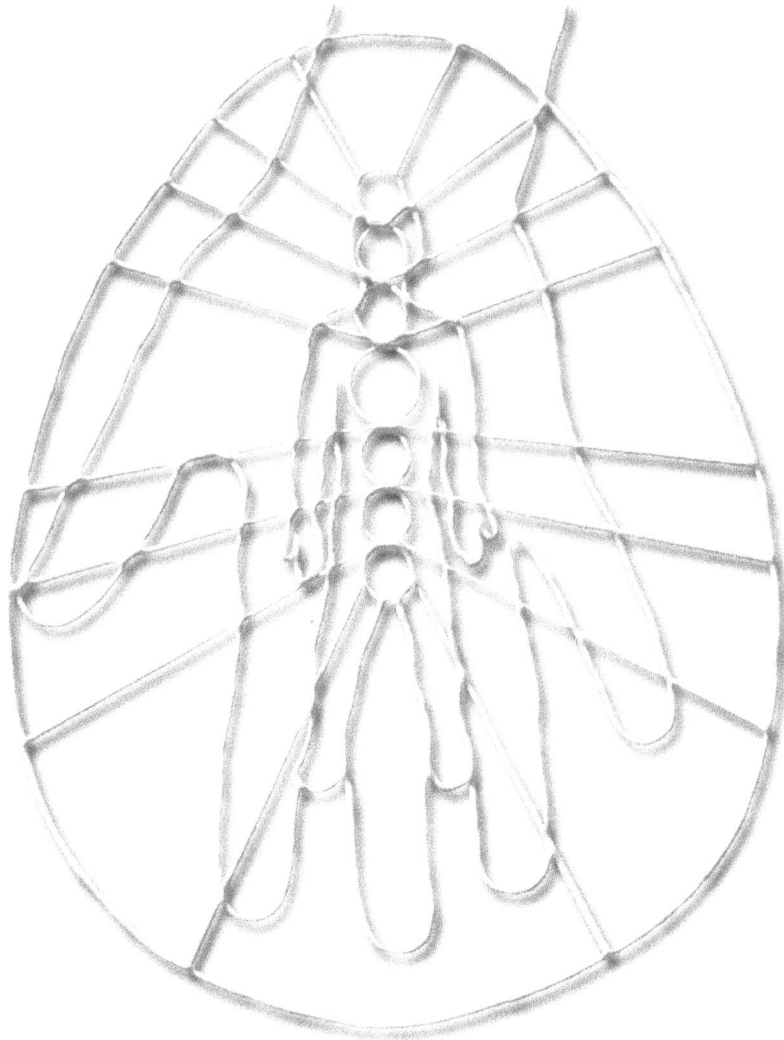

The above design was drawn for the original cover of *Rebirthing According to Spirit* in the early 1980s, now reprinted as Part Two of this book. It is meant to signify an Essene Rebirth, as described in the previous chapters. The egg shape represents the pool of warm water or hot tub. The central figure or "rebirthee" is supported by a large hand, traced from my own hand at the time, which represents the support by the hands of the seven who are there to serve and perform the ritual.

The seven circles represent the seven chakras and the seven AUM chants used in this ritual to activate and spin the chakras. In my original drawing, the circles were done using six dimes and one nickel, with the heart chakra being larger since it is meant to predominate. The rays going out represent the emanations of light that penetrate all and bless all during this ritual.

In the period of time after this ritual was released, we performed many of them by simply having someone recite the instructions given here in Chapters 11 and 12. My hope is that you find the right group of people and the right circumstances to perform this miraculous ritual for yourselves, in commemoration of a time on Earth when the divine was honored as flowing through every aspect of life. The ancient healing temples have been described for you here. The sacred elements of breath, light, sound, and water can indeed be used as "pranic carriers" to bring healing and holiness to the lower bodies of humans and to the Earth herself. ▪

—Denis Ouellette • 2019

PART THREE • **Breakthroughs!**

PART THREE will give you a deeper understanding of Integral Breathwork—the hows and whys of combining good physiological breathing with breathwork, and the benefits that can result. Breakthroughs come in many shapes and sizes, and we offer people several ways to have these—if and when they want them. The stories that follow describe some vivid breakthroughs.

A breakthrough can be achieved by changing how we think of ourselves and our situations. Taking full responsibility for everything in our world can transform us from victim to master. This starts with recognizing the need for change and having a willingness to forgive and move on. It may take courage to embrace the past in order to alter the future. Change may involve the determination to open yourself to natural healing methods and/or the power of grace. It usually involves intent, trust, and courage. We start with the intent to change; then we trust that the healing process can make things better; then we muster the courage to act and sustain the effort until a breakthrough is reached. The French root for *courage* is *coeur,* which means "heart." We define courage as "the coming of age of the heart."

The stories chronicled here are people's peak experiences. These may have come right away or may have taken several sessions to build up to. Not all breakthroughs are dramatic. When people come out of breathwork simply feeling refreshed and content, they've had a good session and learned how to improve their life. Not all breakthroughs are pleasant. Some sessions can be messy. People can become very cold, or hot and sweaty as their nervous system adjusts itself. People can weep or laugh or do both. They may glimpse heaven or look into what has been for them a personal hell. In the next section, you'll read discussions on how to work with people who come to breathwork with a more than ordinary share of burdens, or with blocked energy. Some may have uncomfortable reactions or difficulty integrating their experiences. Great care is taken to bring them back to their center before they leave our six-hour seminar, and follow-up is done when needed. I am grateful to include in this section perspectives from some of the world's foremost breathworkers.

You will read about physical and emotional healings, spontaneous regressions, extrasensory encounters, and spiritual experiences, but breathwork may involve all or none of these for you. Whatever happens will depend on what you and your body are ready for on that day. And if some discomfort comes up, great victories can still be gained from it and profound lessons learned.

As you'll see from our promotional material in the Appendix, the Integral Breathwork seminars are presented from a secular, better-breathing-for-health perspective. This allows people from all walks of life, and from all religious persuasions or none, to feel comfortable coming to this work. Those who recount spiritual experiences during breathwork are those who bring to this work their own understanding of spiritual dimensions. Integral Breathwork starts with correcting the breathing pattern. It is used for self-clearing, oxygenating, detoxing, and energizing. It can be approached purely physiologically; and significant breakthroughs can and do happen just there. Or, people may add their intent to invite spirit into the process in whatever way works for them.

The energy that flows in with the breath—and with the light, the sound, and the water—will follow their thoughts, enhance their aspirations, and strengthen their beliefs. When spirit heals, she is considerate. She doesn't barge in. She waits to be called, she comes in increments, and she takes on the form each person is most comfortable with. ◼

A New Beginning for Me

Nancy O. • Montreal, Canada

Good morning, Rukhs!* I want to say a huge thanks to you for all the preparation you put in for the extraordinary day I had yesterday. For me, I can only say, BREAKTHROUGH and MORE BREAKTHROUGHS! As draining as my experience felt yesterday, the message I got was RELEASE! I was surrounded by wonderful people and felt so safe, even at times when I was feeling much fear. Every facilitator shared a soothing energy, which brought me to my BREAKTHROUGH.

Today, there is still much processing going on for me, and I decided to just let it flow. Then this magnificent energy happened. The person I was talking about yesterday in the discussion circle was my husband. He is the person I've allowed to create all my hurt, pain and anger, which I expressed in my breakthrough. I shared how I went through the pain and then let it go, telling myself that I will no longer accept to live in the fear of his bad behavior towards me, etc. (He has always been extremely restrictive. I even had to get his signature on the check I wrote for coming to this seminar.)

Well, this morning, when a regular morning with him is always stressful, with his anger and aggression, SOMETHING ENTIRELY DIFFERENT was going on in our interaction. He felt that something was different this morning; I could see it in his eyes. He knew I wasn't afraid of him anymore, because I looked at him straight in his eyes as he spoke to me. He could no longer use his controlling ways on me, which left him weak and lost. He had no choice but to surrender, and then he was very calm and respectful.

This is without even telling him anything about my experiences yesterday—my energy expressed it all to him. He felt that the power and control he had over me, and how he could belittle me and scare me, was not going to work anymore. He felt my strong energy this morning—I know he did! His attitude sent me a thousand messages.

I feel WONDERFUL about this! I feel like I just got out of jail and am able to live my freedom again. I feel like I am able to be me again.

I wanted you to know how much Denis and everyone helped me in my transformation into My Authentic Self—my ultimate goal in my life right now... I have to create a new life now for me. There are no limits to what I feel I can do now, with so much of my fear lifted off. A new beginning for me...

THANKS SO MUCH! XO

Special thanks to my dearest friends, Rukhshana Surty, B.Ed., RMT, and her husband Ian Ramsey, B.A., BSc., Dip.Ed., for sponsoring me several times at their yoga center in Montreal to come for weekend trainings, which included private bodywork/breathwork sessions as well. Find them at: Recess-From-Stress.com. I am also pleased that the Integral Breathwork torch is passed to the next generation, in the person of Katie McIntyre, who also sponsored me in Montreal for additional trainings. She carries on her wonderful practice via: MindBodyMontreal.com.

Young Indian Brave

Denis Ouellette • San Diego, CA

Cochise starts off his first discourse with the words, "Through the waters of your subconscious and into the conscious mind, you have come at this time." The Medicine Way has always been steeped in symbols, dreams, and the mysteries of nature and the spirit world. Shamans talk about "soul retrieval," finding and restoring vital energy lost due to a traumatic event. Cochise says in the text that breathwork may be combined with regression, even into past lives, and hypnosis. I do recommend that these practices be left to trained professionals. I do feel one should not go looking out of mere curiosity into areas of the mind that are locked away for a good reason. And I would also think twice about letting another person put suggestions into my subconscious mind.

Yet sometimes a revelation comes out of the past for the purpose of healing. This is one such story of a young sailor who served with me in the late '70s on the USS *Sperry* at the Point Loma submarine base in San Diego. Andrew was in his early twenties and a typical sailor except for his ornery nature. He bucked authority and seemed to go around with a certain peevishness all the time. I thought I might be able to help him. I knew Andrew had Native American blood in him, and as I had an audiotape of Cochise guiding a meditation for finding one's unique spirit animal, I invited Andrew to do the meditation. He agreed. To take Andrew into a receptive state, Cochise used some rhythmic breathing and a classic hypnosis countdown.

But before Andrew could get into discovering his spirit animal, he was off into his own world, where dramatic events were taking place. He was totally involved, as if watching a vivid movie, and it was a bit hard to draw the details out of him, but he was apparently seeing a past life as a young Indian brave, probably about his same age. He was in the wilds somewhere out West, and two older white men were harassing him. They had cornered him and his horse along the edge of a cliff. There was some jostling. Suddenly, out of pure spite and cruelty, they pushed his horse over the cliff to its death. Then they rode away, stranding him to walk back to his camp alone.

It was apparent from Andrew's stunned reaction what pain this caused him, and how much he had loved his horse. Reliving all this now, he was in tears. I managed to suggest, "See your horse in the sky now, running free in the clouds." Apparently this helped, because he asked, "Can I ride him?" He saw himself riding his beloved friend once again.

The scene shifted and now, he was in the woods, spying on the campfire circle of a neighboring tribe. He spotted for the first time a young Indian maiden, the daughter of the chief, the most beautiful creature he had ever seen. He was experiencing his first flush of young love.

That was about it. We went to bed in our berths below decks. The next morning, Andrew told me he had dreamt the rest of the story. He had gone on to marry that young maiden and had become chief of his tribe. He never forgave the white men for their cruelty, and he carried hatred for all white men to the end of that life.

And apparently into this life, until the memory could be brought back for understanding and resolving. About six months later, I picked Andrew up hitchhiking on Point Loma. He was wearing a brightly colored polyester shirt—this was the '70s, after all! He had found a girlfriend, and life was going well for him. ▪

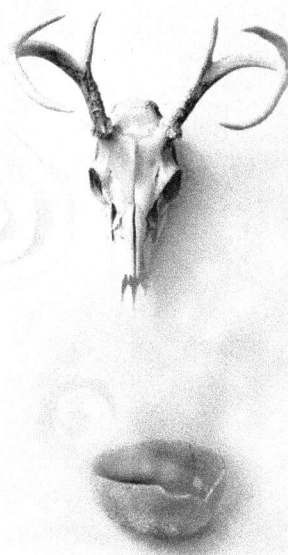

Who Is That? Is That You?

Joan Belle Nemeth • Billings, MT

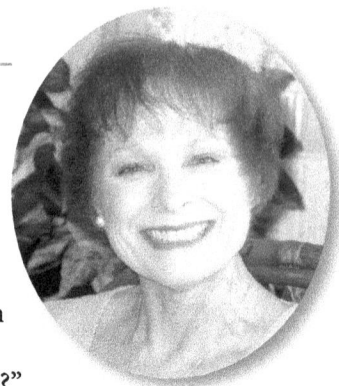

When people see a picture of me taken two or more years ago, they often ask me, "Who is that? Is that you?" They wonder, "What have you been doing?" Occasionally I get, "Do I know you?" from people who haven't seen me in a while. When they recognize my voice again, I hear, "Joan? Is that you?" About two years ago, I set myself on a path of self-healing. Breathwork has been a major contributor to my health and happiness. It has literally breathed new life and a new outlook into me and added new dimension to what I understood as wholeness.

I was born into a family where a healthy lifestyle was encouraged, mainly by my U.S. Army father. My father was the son of Hungarian immigrants, and as a boy, he had suffered with bouts of pneumonia and was sickly. As an adult, he determined to do all he could to stay healthy. Unfortunately, he died at the age of 63 after succumbing to injuries from Vietnam, injuries that would likely have killed him sooner than the eight years he lived after the war had it not been for his healthy lifestyle. In my own search for healing, I came to appreciate his adherence to natural methods only after an arduous detour through the medical system. At least I learned firsthand what worked for me and what definitely did not. Because of my father, I was always open to trying what was simple, meaningful and practical. If he were alive today, he would be right here with me enjoying breathwork.

Was there to be only one way for me to attain greater health? Not hardly! My pursuit of wellness has been multifaceted, and I've always stayed open to what presents itself. I too had childhood pneumonia, and somewhere in our travels abroad, I was exposed to tuberculosis. I further injured my lungs in a chlorine-gas-inhalation accident in my high-school chemistry lab. On several occasions, for various reasons, I climbed on the pharmaceutical merry-go-round. One reason was my intense fight with asthma, beginning at age 33. This five-year battle for breath included pneumonia three times and bronchitis almost constantly! During the fifth year, there was only one month when I was *not* on antibiotics, steroids, or other drugs. It was becoming clear to me that relying on drugs was a big mistake.

At my doctor's suggestion, I began taking weekly allergy shots and did so for the next five years. I endured that ordeal until the needles could no longer penetrate the tissues in my arms. Did those shots improve my lung capacity to a point of sustainable wellness? No, they did not. I did stop coughing, and that was a relief, but I would not fully understand how much healthier my life could be until I determined there would be no more medications and no more shots! Always present was the lingering worry that my lungs would not be capable of sustaining health, so how could I change that? My move to Montana helped immeasurably, as this finally put me in touch with alternative healing choices I could embrace.

I discovered breathwork on the chance recommendation of my dance instructor. She had attended a breathwork seminar led by Denis, and had found it instructive and helpful. Knowing my lungs were in need of any help they could get, I thought this might be a useful, drugless tool. What could be more basic than breathing—the pure and simple technique of bringing oxygen into your body and detoxing it through the exhale!

After all I had been through, could it really be this simple? I only had to let go and trust my body's ability to heal itself. I listened to and observed how my body was working and allowed myself to breathe in new life within the caring and competent atmosphere created at these seminars. Each session was different and offered me a new experience of self-discovery. My first session was sheer bliss as fresh oxygen circulated throughout my blood. As I sat up after that first time, you couldn't have wiped the smile off my face if you tried!

During my fourth session, I felt the release of physical cellular memories from old injuries to my neck, knee, and ankle all at once. I had the feeling that I was being yanked by the head* and also by the leg and foot. It was breath-stoppingly painful for a few moments, but I just kept on breathing! It was as though the breathing allowed me to relive and then let go of that hurt. My ninth session left me awash with a sense of personal wonder and renewal.

My regular use of breathwork has brought my lungs to their full capacity. I have continued to study Integral Breathwork and now assist at the seminars. My experiences are a rare and wonderful gift. In one session, I assisted a woman who, even though she was sitting up, held her head down and did not appear to be breathing. I knelt behind her and asked her to lean onto me. I spoke quietly to her to take in my breath. For a few minutes, I had the sensation that my breath was somehow entering her body. It felt as though I was literally breathing for both of us. Slowly, she began to breathe with me on her own and eventually relaxed into her own rhythm. Later she told me, "You gave me a reason to live." A powerful statement from someone you thought you were just helping with breathwork!

I am grateful for how I have changed and how I'll keep on changing. I understand more deeply who I am and my purpose in life. My practice is in psycho-structural balancing, neuromuscular therapy, and other modalities. I encourage my clients to incorporate breathwork to achieve body-mind wholeness. To say it all in one sentence, *breathe and be well!*

*A physical sensation often associated with the release of a birth trauma.

They Were OK

Rocky Larocco, Emergency Medical Technician (EMT) & Firefighter • Bozeman, MT

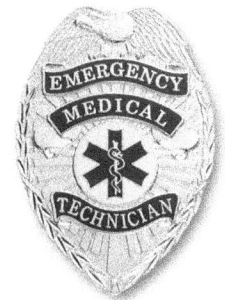

I have done two breathwork seminars. The workshops are really great, but my first one was incredible. When we got to the breathing part of the session, I experienced something I did not expect. As I got more into the breathing, I really felt like I started to soar up and out of my body. I could actually look down on my body laying there breathing.

Then, somewhere in this, I started seeing people who had died in car accidents whose lives I had attempted to save in my work as a firefighter and EMT. It was not a bad thing; it was like they where telling me they were OK and that I did my best to save them. I have struggled with this and have experienced post traumatic stress syndrome because of it. After seeing their faces and hearing they were OK, it was easier for me to go back out on calls.

During that same session, I had contact with two friends of mine who had died of cancer. They also let me know they were OK. It was really incredible. I've never experienced anything quite like this before, and I am grateful that I did.

I also learned how to help people use their breathing to get through the trauma of a car accident or injury.

Thanks!

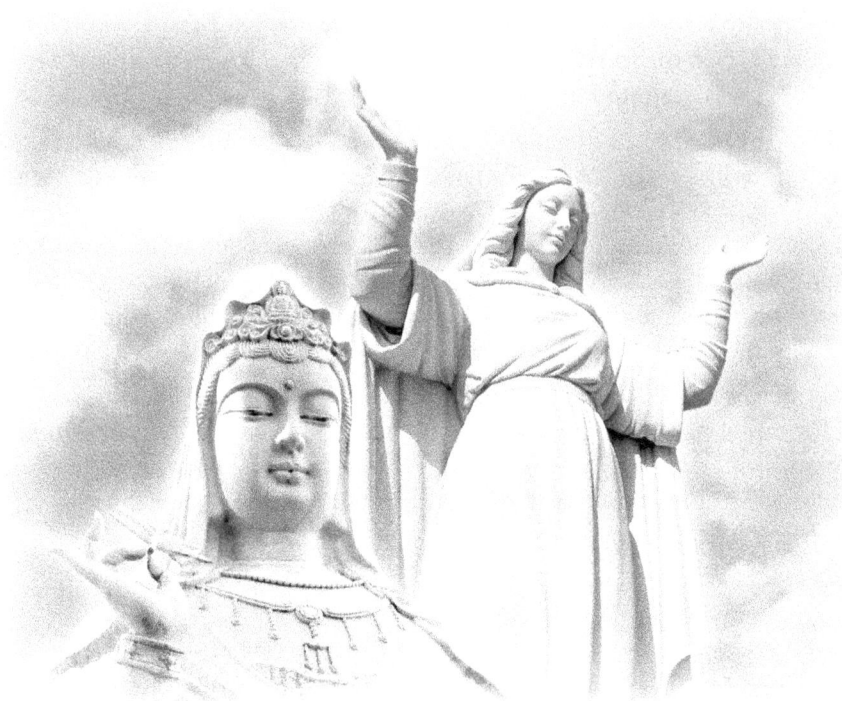

Adele's Communion

Adele Tate • Helena, MT

When I read the manuscript for Part Two of this book, I couldn't put it down. Finally, I was reading about my cherished dream of rebuilding the healing temples I remembered in my soul from ancient times.

For more than two decades, I have studied how touch influences the energy of the cells in the body. In equine massage, I discovered that horses can't learn if they are in pain. Working an area of pain in a clockwise direction activates father energy, which strengthens the area. Working in a counter-clockwise direction activates mother energy to draw out pain and toxins while nurturing and supporting. This was my first awareness of energy healing.

Years later, I went to China to learn Qigong, the study of raising energies from the earth (mother) and pulling them from the sky (father) to direct them into every cell of the body. Qigong balances these yin-yang energies. Recently, I have been trained in Foot Zone Balance. By using these same clockwise and counter-clockwise movements, a "footzonologist" can activate the DNA within each cell. By regular zoning of the feet, and through breathwork and other natural therapies, you can transform yourself by reconnecting with your original blueprint stored within the cellular DNA.

In the past, I worked with other groups of healers who used the breath to reach levels of meditation that were instructive, clearing, and healing, but the Integral Breathwork system is the most effective I have experienced.

During one of my breathwork sessions, my goal was to heal an old break in my hip. As I began to breathe, a strong vibration moved up my body to the hip area, and I felt all my bones were vibrating at a very high rate. As I continued to breathe, my hips released. I allowed my knees to open and placed the bottoms of my feet together. There was a shift in the hip joint and an intense vibration in the area of the break. I prayed to Mother Mary and Kuan Yin for compassion. Within seconds, two facilitators took my hands and sent so much love to my heart that I couldn't hold it. I wept with gratitude. My inner voice told me that I am perfect and that God wishes me to see only my perfection.

❖—❖ ❖—❖ ❖—❖

*[The following is an excerpt from Adele's letter to me after one seminar.
Adele's experience shows how sometimes a synergy occurs
between the participants in a session. —Editor]*

This last session was the most gentle I have had so far. The goal-setting process was somewhat emotional for me, but then the breathing itself was fairly effortless and gentle. I usually *work* as though I not only have to get up the hill, but I have to be the first one to the top! I didn't have to achieve that intense vibration that I usually strive for. Mother Mary and Kuan Yin were holding me in a great white aura.

A very gentle vibration started at my feet and slowly moved up to the heart chakra, then continued up the spine to the cranium. There seemed to be a stuck place there. A facilitator placed his fingers on the occipital bones and said, "Give this to me." I panicked for a second and then released my shoulders. The vibration moved over the top of my head and flowed into my heart chakra. I felt restored and balanced. Shafts of white and gold energy emanated from my hands to the other participants. I felt a comforting energy reach someone who was crying across the room.

Earlier, during the goal setting, I had stated, "I'm terrified of losing my dad!" Since my mother's passing in December, I panic whenever my dad says he isn't feeling well or when he's feeling lonely. As I lay there continuing to breathe, I heard the sound of a powerful vibration enveloping me. I watched as my winged pegasus scooped me up, and we flew into the universe. I found myself at the throne of my heavenly Father. He took me into his loving arms and assured me that I would never lose Him, that He loved me and *accepted* me to Himself. I wondered at the meaning of this word. I repeated it several times as I came back into my body and the vibrations subsided. I was complete. Communion with the Father had healed my worries for my earthly father.

I am grateful to my dearest healing friends for these experiences. ▨

Let Go and Forgive

T.C.V. • Helena, MT

I love breathwork. It has its own innate intelligence that can do deep healing and release work exactly where you need it. I feel that setting your intentions before your session is very important. I knew I had been sexually molested as a very young child, at about age two, and I went into my first breathwork with the intention of healing this in myself. It was work for me at first to keep the pace, to ride the breathwork bicycle uphill, but I did.

Then I was gone to this world. I regressed to being a tiny toddler dealing with various emotions of abuse, mostly sadness. I was able to forgive my molesters. Then that episode seemed to be gone and my body tension and breathing relaxed for a little while.

Then I was gone again, regressed into a past-life memory of being raped. I was a hungry Russian girl in my twenties. Hoping to find some food, I entered a building where some Russian soldiers were having a party. I was wearing lots of bulky clothes and a coat because it was very cold outside. I hid in the cloakroom, trying to figure out how to get the food, but five soldiers found me there and raped me. During the breathwork, I was struggling to push them away. I was yelling, "Get them off of me! I want them off me, far away from me, even their spirits! They have no right!"

By some grace, reviewing both of these events has helped me to resolve the emotional charge and freed me to see sexuality more as a loving act, and myself more as a lover instead of an object of sexual lust. This, of course, has helped me relax and enjoy life more.

After this session, I talked to a psychic friend and told her I felt I needed more work on releasing my past. She looked at my aura and said, "You don't need any more releasing from this lifetime, but you still need releasing from past lives."

Four months later, when the breathworkers came to town again, my intention was to understand why I am such a hoarder and why I have trouble believing in abundance. It seems that I believe I never have enough. My session was full of very deep sadness and crying. Again, I was gone from this world, and I regressed into being a German Jewish woman in my thirties. My Jewish husband and I and our two daughters, ages nine and eleven, were locked away in a small German concentration camp where we were separated. I was put in with other women. We lived in outdoor cages made of barbed wire. We were starving.

The young German guards, mostly in their early twenties, looked horrified. If they went against regulations, they would also have been killed. Once in a while, they tried to sneak us extra food. I felt they could be my sons. I did not feel like a victim or that they were my predators. I felt we were all in this tragedy together, playing different roles—we had a oneness with each other. However, I still had to forgive the Nazi political machine and all of those involved in it.

Before I died of starvation, I felt that if we had lived far away in the country with lots of stored food and supplies, we wouldn't have been found by the Nazis and taken to this concentration camp to die. Now, in this lifetime, with my husband and my two daughters, I live in the country away from view, with lots of stored food, blankets, warm clothes, books, and games.

Unconsciously holding on to the fear of starvation from that life, I felt a need to protect myself and my loved ones in this life. The breathwork has taught me that the best thing to do with past fear is to let it go and to forgive. I feel less fearful now, and happier. I no longer feel the old urge to hoard food for later. I feel I can accept my abundance more serenely. The word *government* also seems easier to say without so many negative connotations.

I am grateful and thankful for this breathwork. I love how it seems to know exactly what to do to release the past and make my life more whole and joyful. I feel that I am no longer living my life as just a reaction to the past, but am able to live more in the moment.

I am most grateful to the breathwork facilitators. I know that I could not do this work without their completely loving support and assistance. They are like angels to me. I also appreciate the understanding of good physical breathing they taught me. Now, many times throughout the day, I remember to breathe deeply into my tummy. This seems to melt small stresses away. I was also grateful for the abundant fruit feast we shared at the end of the seminar that seemed to appear out of nowhere. It felt like I was in heaven already.

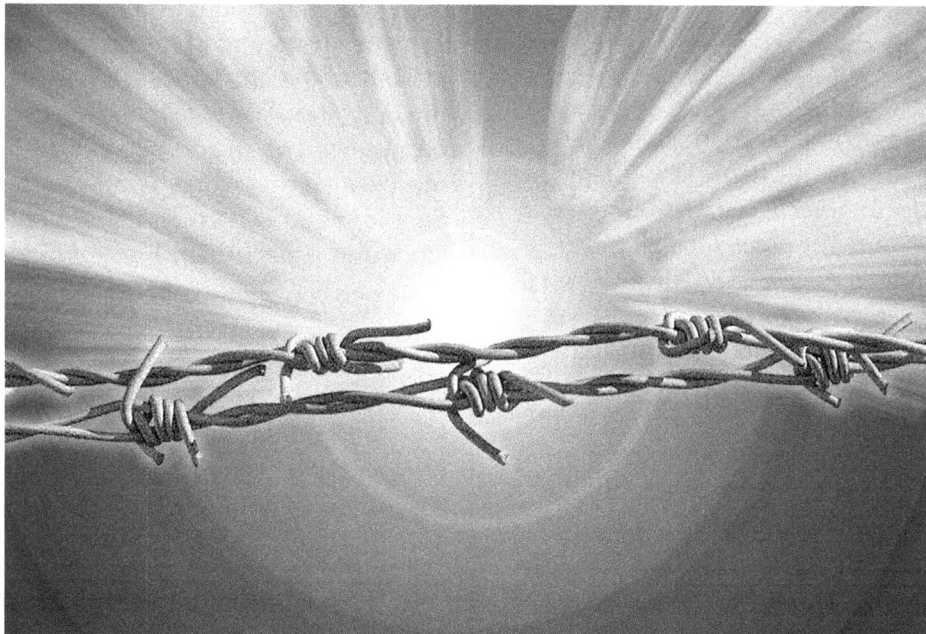

An Ode to Massage

Lessons from a Lifetime of Body Tune-Ups

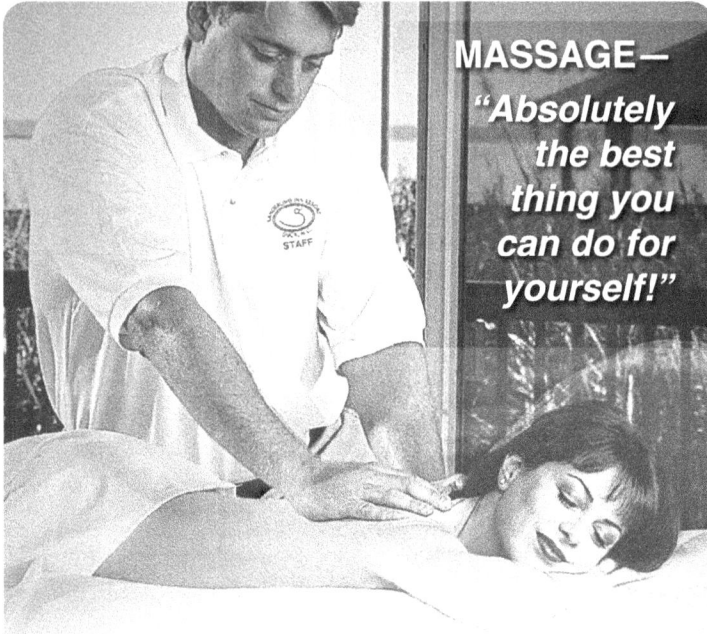

MASSAGE—
"Absolutely the best thing you can do for yourself!"

Denis Ouellette, LMT, OBDS

After a tune-up and oil change, you say things to your mechanic like: *"Great, I'm good for another 3000 miles." "She's really hummin' now!"* and *"My acceleration is much better."* Well, after a good BODY TUNE-UP, you'll be saying similar things to your therapist! We wouldn't think of NOT doing regular maintenance and repairs on our precious motor vehicle... running it low on oil, or driving it with low air in the tires. But how many miles have you put on your BODY since its last tune-up?

The first Model-T rolled off Henry Ford's assembly line in 1913, and today we know a lot about cars. How ancient is the human body— back to Adam and Eve? Still today, how much do we really understand about our far more precious body systems? Yes, we know that a great massage soothes sore muscles and creates relaxation, but it can do so much more. **Let's take a look under the hood.**

1) The MUSCLES & BODY STRUCTURE

In a good massage, we usually address the hurtingest body parts first, but you'll notice there's some muscle pain you know about, and some you don't—until we start digging around a bit.

Just about everyone comes in wanting their shoulders, upper back, low back, and neck worked on. And we do address those areas to get relief. But as we progress, the client will report pain in areas of chronic tension they didn't know they had. Typically these hide in the lats (upper sides of the back), in the glutes (deep in the upper butt and hip-joint areas (where low-back pain can usually be traced back to), the IT bands (outer sides of the legs, especially up by the hips), the insides of the calf muscles near the knees, and in the quads (strong muscles in front, above the knees). Pain in the front of the delt (shoulder cap) muscle is usually more pronounced on the dominant side. This is a muscle area that works awfully hard for most people, whether it's physical labor or computer work, and it will usually present hidden pain.

Once you start exploring, though, *oh!*—can these areas reveal what they've been storing. The good news is that, with just the right bodywork and breathwork, they CAN be released, and this will free up a lot of energy. Chronically tense muscles and other blockages are robbing you of energy in the background.

The wonderful thing about the body is that, if we can just get 10–20% of these hot spots (trigger points) relieved, then 80–90% of the pain can go away.

Good therapy just stays there, patiently working on those key spots until true release happens. There's no rush... and you CAN communicate with these muscles, through the nervous system and breathing. With just the right amount of pressure and various techniques, they will finally let go of even YEARS of accumulated tension, waste buildup, structural dysfunction, etc... *So, when did you say your last tune-up was?*

When you get a massage and loosen up much of your muscle tension BEFORE a chiropractic adjustment, then there's a better chance, FIRST, that the bony structure, especially along the spine, will respond and cooperate, and SECOND, that the adjustments will last, because that chronic-tension pattern will not be there to pull that vertebra or bone back out of place. Long-term resolution of injury, misalignment, or strain involves addressing a combination of symptoms and systems holistically.

2) The BREATHING & NERVOUS SYSTEMS This familiar face belongs to Dr. Andrew Weil, one of the pioneers of holistic health in this country. This is his CD course, ***Breathing, The Master Key to Self Healing.*** As a young doctor, he traveled to the Far East. He thought he'd be learning about exotic diseases, like *tsetse fly sleeping sickness*, but what do you suppose he discovered were the #1 most prevalent disorders and diseases? It was issues related to stress and anxiety.

He brought back and introduced to Western medicine a better understanding of the **Autonomic Nervous System (ANS).** This system governs ALL of your INTERNAL functions, most notably your digestion, glands and hormones, heart rate, and immune function. Your internal nerves are immediately sensitive to any stress triggers *(real or imagined)*. When you go into "fight-or-flight," digestion shuts down, as does the functioning of the immune system. Stress hormones get released: *"I can't fight germs right now; I'm running from a bear!"*

Dr. Weil teaches that there's only one effective entryway into the influencing of the ANS and calming it down—and that's through **conscious breathing.** All great bodywork includes breathwork.

A breath-savvy therapist will help you correct and improve any dysfunctions they discover (such as predominantly high-chest breathing). Every time the therapist moves into a painful area, it will be accompanied by a wonderful exhale, as in—***Hhaaaaaaawwwwww!*** (Otherwise, the ANS interprets this as INVASIVE pain, which will trigger a counterproductive stress response.) Just as in yoga, along with every good stretch comes a good, deep breath.

For best results, every letting go of pain must also be a letting go, through the breath and the ANS, of the inner patterns of thought and feeling, and a releasing of the cellular, nerve, and muscle memories of the original trauma.

3) The IMMUNE, LYMPH & DIGESTIVE SYSTEMS We've all heard the buzzwords for the sympathetic, stress response side of the ANS as "fight-or-flight." The buzzwords for when the body finally arrives to the parasympathetic side of the ANS are "rest, digest and heal." These three goals simply cannot be achieved when a person is stuck in "fight-or-flight," and unfortunately, for most of us—that's MOST of the time! That's our modern-day *tsetse-fly* dilemma. *A good body tune-up can get you there!*

The therapist will also be on the lookout for another "weirdish" kind of pain that's usually associated with stagnation and blockage of the lymph system. It is usually found in places like along the insides of the shinbones, and on the

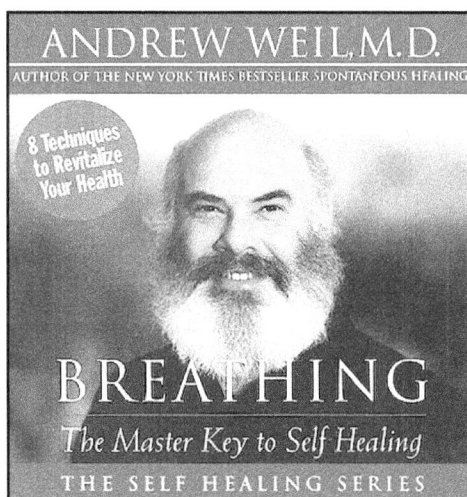

ANDREW WEIL, M.D.
AUTHOR OF THE NEW YORK TIMES BESTSELLER SPONTANEOUS HEALING

8 Techniques to Revitalize Your Health

BREATHING
The Master Key to Self Healing
THE SELF HEALING SERIES

webs between the toes, but mainly behind the pec muscles near the armpits (see baby).

The lymph system is the body's water-based, waste-removal system that lies just under the skin. Stagnant lymph is like "leaves from last fall still stuck in your rain-gutters." The therapist will get all that moving again, and this will prevent a world of problems later on.

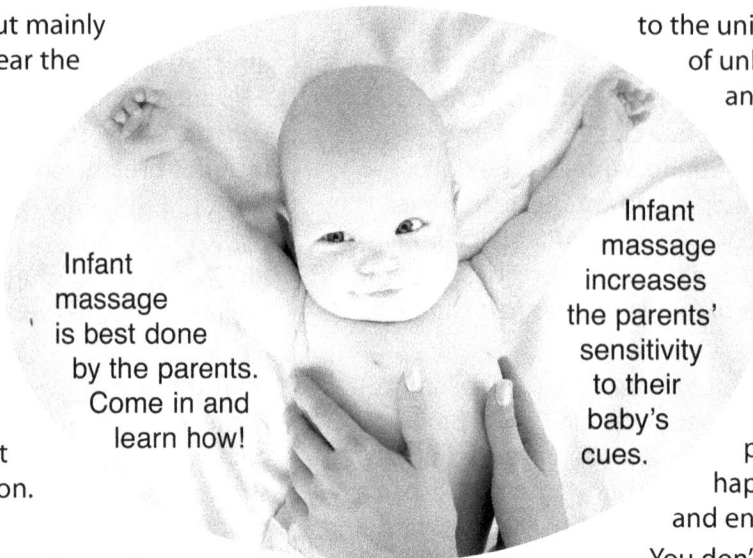

Infant massage is best done by the parents. Come in and learn how!

Infant massage increases the parents' sensitivity to their baby's cues.

to the universal source of unlimited power and energy, and letting THAT move in, through and around the session, leaving both therapist and client happy, filled up, and energized.

You don't have to see the wind to perceive its effects. You don't have to *understand* energy work, but you can still respect it, acknowledge it, invoke it, and allow it to do its perfect work alongside of you. Again, breathing work is the #1 facilitator of energy movement. Oxygen (inhaling) is our #1 source of fuel. Exhaling is our #1 means of detoxification.

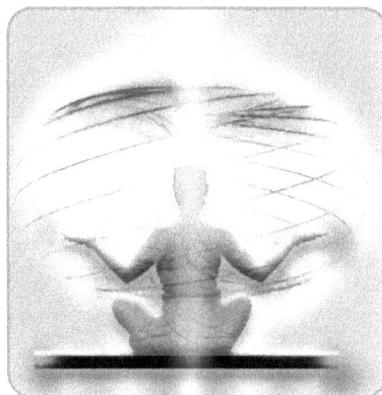

4) The ENERGY SYSTEM Energy is a funny thing because it's always everywhere and influencing everything, but also invisible and not paid much attention to. Energy exchanges happen all the time—with a smile (or a frown), with every word we say, and along with the lightest touch. A lot of energy-flow happens in a massage, especially when there is copious breathing going on.

We can think of energy as the animating life-force of the universe. It goes on *"within you and without you,"* to quote George Harrison. In massage, no matter what modality they practice, good therapists will be LESS concerned about the energy exchange between client and therapist (in either direction) and MORE concerned about connecting

5) STRETCHING & MOVEMENT

A good session includes a lot of great stretches and most of them will be super-slow. When you take a lot of time to pull an arm, or both legs, for example, it gives NOT ONLY the muscles and nerves, at the cellular level, a chance to open up and relieve constrictions, BUT ALSO the fascia—the body's superstructure, which will always resist quick,

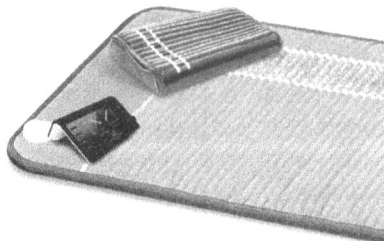

"herky-jerky" stretches.

When stretches and other flowing movements (*effleurage*) are done super-slowly, as when pressing upward along the spinal muscles, then the nervous system can predict the movement and cooperate in its communication to the muscles, allowing them to TRULY let go. Increased range of motion (without pain) and more ease of movement are the immediate, evident results of a good massage.

6) The BIOMAT (See ad opposite page.) The far-infrared heat coming from this highly advanced heating pad penetrates 6–8 inches into the body and heats muscles and organs through and through.

The mat also emits negative ions, like those that appear after a thunderstorm, or in the presence of a waterfall. The extensive research on the benefits of this mat shows that warming the body like this activates dormant enzymes (the biocatalysts of the body). And at the high-heat setting, they say it even kills cancer cells. This luxurious heat, through amethyst crystals, truly melts away tension on several levels. Clients say that lying on the Biomat alone is worth the price of admission.

So, what can YOU expect from a 60- or 90-minute body tune-up? Well, like the mechanic says: *a better hum in your engine, less wear and tear, and better mileage overall.* And with continued maintenance, you can enjoy a longer life and a healthier, more trouble-free vehicle.

Giving all your body systems a rest and a reset can change the whole trajectory of your outlook on life. Yes, the muscles are the obvious beneficiaries, and they will be happier and freer, but their OWNER gets to move through life without all that accumulated stress. The ripple effect of that is far-reaching. A body tune-up is the best thing you can do for yourself—*get yours today!* ∎

Denis Ouellette, OBDS, LMT, *has been doing bodywork and breathwork for 25+ years. He works out of his studio in Livingston and in Bozeman at Able Chiropractic and Wellness WORx.*

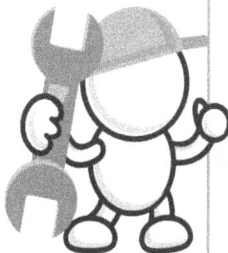

Tips for Bodyworkers

1) Incorporate breathing seamlessly into everything you do.

Both clients and therapists get tired of: "Take a deep breath!" Instead, build breathing phrases into your language, such as: "I'm going to give you a good push here the next time you breathe out." Any potentially painful pressure should be accompanied by an exhale. This counteracts the defensive, "fight-or-flight" response that pain usually elicits. Other phrases I find myself using are: "Breath right here..." or "Give me a Hhuuuuuuuuh." If you're on a trigger point, such as on the trapezius or in the glute, wait for that slack-jawed, relaxed exhale, and then push inward. Modulate the pressure so that relaxation is maintained.

2) Be such a great breather yourself that it becomes contagious.

Become a "breather" yourself first! This may take 6 to 10 breathwork sessions before all stuck breathing patterns are removed from your own system. You will notice an immediate breath from the belly happening, without conscious thought, whenever something stressful comes up. Congratulations! Now, surround your clients with that sound. Breathing louder than them every time gives them the freedom to open up their own patterns.

3) How to coach someone's breathing.

It's usually in the second half for me, when they've rolled over and are on their back. Ask them to place their hands on their lower belly. "OK, lower still, with your pinkies almost on your hip bones." Ask for a deep breath. If you get a chest breath, coach them to start it off in their belly. They may be either a "feeling" or a "visual" person, or both. Place the back of their hand on your lower belly—the front of their hand is a bit too personal—and/or say, "Watch my belly." Then show them a great diaphragmatic inhale. If they do it, say, "Good!" (Praise them to no end when they do anything well.) OK to breathe into the ribs and chest secondarily and thirdly.

4) What to do if a *bona fide* breathwork session starts to happen.

When a person is new to deep breathing, they may enter into the tingling of the hands or other sensations. Tell them they're going into a breathwork session, but depending on time and the situation, simply scale it down. Discuss with them doing a REAL breathwork session at some other time, with better preparation on what to do and what to expect. Relate the major benefits of breathwork. ▪

Tetany & Gentle Breathwork

Denis Ouellette & Michael Grant White

with perspectives by Leon Chaitow & Tom Goode

Denis Ouellette:

One of the most daunting and least understood aspects of breathwork is the muscle cramping (tetany) that can occur especially in the first few sessions. It begins as tingling, mostly in the hands and sometimes in the feet or mouth area. These muscles may then retract and become stiff for a brief cycle, about 15 minutes—but this can seem like hours for the breather. In our experience with the Integral Breathwork system, tetany occurs mildly in about 10% of the initial sessions, more acutely in about 3% of initial sessions, and only intermittently thereafter. In other forms of breathwork where high-chest breathing is stressed, for instance, I've seen the percentages much higher.

Assistance from the breathworker is helpful to guide the breather through this. Gentle massage can be relieving. I often gently, yet fully, extend the palm at the wrist, along with all five fingers, backward against the inward reflex of the stiffening (see photo opposite page). I will time this backward movement with an exhale. We've found that the *Zap-A-Kramp* herbal pillows [see ad in Resources], which contain common club moss, work well to relieve the cramping, while the tingling will remain until it cycles through. Having the breather slow down on the exhale has a calming effect. This makes sense physiologically, as Mike White will describe below.

In the early days, when tetany came about during a session people used to say, "Oh, you're resisting," as if there were a fear-based conscious or subconscious basis to it. I see it rather as a temporary overload in the releasing process because of *chi* activation and/or cellular-memory release, which can be avoided altogether or worked through effectively, mainly through relaxation.

In Part Two, Chapter 8, John the Divine spoke about the release of cellular memories from the muscles and the cells themselves, and the activation of the body's subconscious mental and emotional aspects. Certainly, there are changes going on here at many levels. I see the tingling as a physically felt, cellular reaction to increased oxygenation, and an energetic upswing in the breather's atomic vibratory frequency. As each new oxygen atom releases its additional electron, things can get moving.

The energetic pathways through the body (the meridians) will conduct this life-force. The exit points for the meridians are at the hands and feet and indeed at the mouth. I have found it helpful to guide clients to visualize their hands as open doorways—exits rather than dead-ends or bottlenecks. As they breathe out, I ask them to see their energy passing through and beyond their fingertips. This, along with more letting go on the exhale (calmer, slower, and more relaxed), allows the tetany to pass more smoothly. More intense and especially high-chest breathing and the onset of tetany itself can cause a sympathetic reaction in the autonomic nervous system, i.e., they can bring on a sense of fear or panic and can bring about an oxygen/carbon dioxide imbalance.

Michael Grant White:

From a physical perspective, this cramping can be viewed as vaso-constriction (constriction of the blood vessels causing the muscles to cramp). An accelerated balanced or unbalanced breathing pattern can create overbreathing or hyperventilation, which results in hypocapnea, a condition of too little carbon dioxide in the blood plasma, causing the oxygen to not be uptaken sufficiently by the red blood cells. This is commonly known as shunting. The over-breathing does not allow carbon dioxide to build up enough for the body to register its increased need for oxygen, so it keeps the gates closed like a river dam holding the water back. This insufficient CO_2 can cause constriction of the blood vessels, muscular contraction, and tension or cramping in the extremities.

My viewpoint is that tetany comes about primarily due to the sympathetic aspect of the breathing pattern (shallow, rapid chest breathing rather than fuller, lower abdominal breathing). The more you breathe in the high chest, the more excitable and overstimulated is the sympathetic response, whereas the more you breathe diaphragmatically through the abdominal areas, the more the system calms down in a parasympathetic response. Even with deeper and larger breaths, which could easily be called overbreathing or hyperventilation, it is possible to not produce tetany. So I conclude that it is not so much the breath rate or volume that is involved, although given deep and fast enough breathing, that could well be, but whether the breathing pattern is predominantly sympathetic or parasympathetic. Breath-workers often find that extending the exhale will produce a backing off of the tetany as the longer, slower exhale allows the body to build up the necessary carbon dioxide.

If the tetany is acute and does not lessen with additional breathwork sessions,

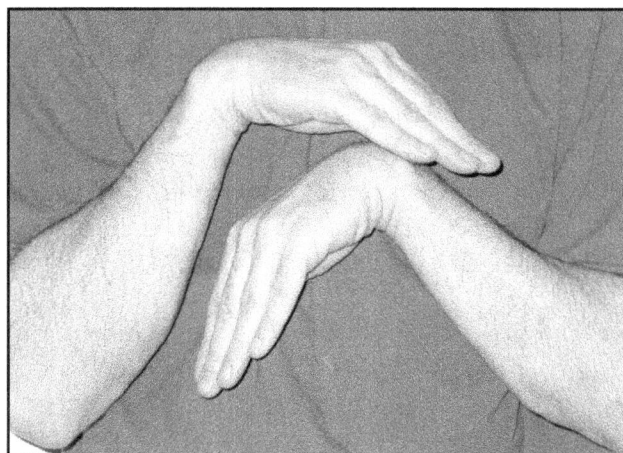

The *Oxford University Atlas of Clinical Neurology* states, "Tetany is caused by the tonic spasm of the intrinsic hand muscles," which means the muscles on the inside of the hand contract, but this doesn't explain why. This article includes several causative reasons as to why this occurs during breathwork and puts forth means to address it. The picture above is the editor's simulation. Tetany usually involves only the hands and wrists. The muscles of the forearms and upper arms may also contract (as shown) but only in more extreme cases. Sometimes the facial muscles, the feet and other muscle groups may be involved.

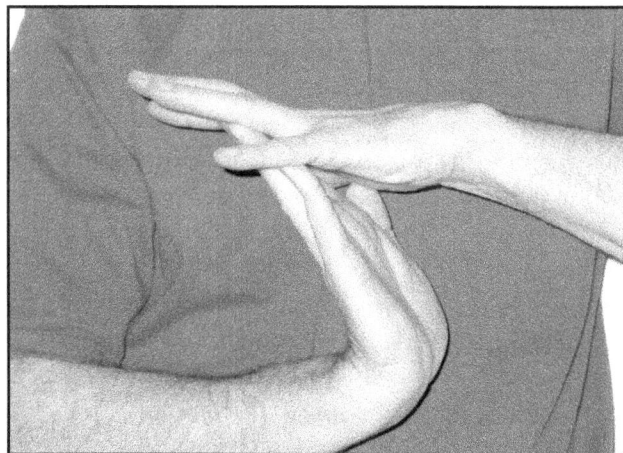

This is one massage technique we use to work with hands stiffened by tetany. On the person's exhale, the facilitator will gently pull back in the reverse direction of the contracted muscles, returning the hands to pause at their contracted state during the inhale. This can be done about 20 times in rhythm with the breath. Facilitators can coach the client to relax and release the hands on the exhale, and to visualize the opening of the hand meridian's exit points as they exhale.

Improper Breathing Patterns

If breathing is more rapid than is ideal for the current needs of the body, we lose too much carbon dioxide and therefore carbonic acid, and the blood becomes more alkaline than normal. This creates a state of respiratory alkalosis: the blood pH moves from a normal of around 7.4 to as much as 7.5. Not much change, you might say, but what a difference it makes! The effects are dramatic. Anxiety appears (and therefore, so does even faster breathing), aggravating the feeling of anxiety or even panic. Smooth muscles constrict. And since these surround all of the "tubes" of the body, this creates a narrowing of the blood vessels and interferes with normal digestion and bladder function. A process known as the Bohrs effect begins, causing the red blood cells to bind more tightly to the oxygen molecules they carry. This means not only less blood gets to the brain and muscles, but also less oxygen is released. This creates profound fatigue and a lack of mental clarity, or "brain fog."

Sympathetic arousal occurs, creating altered neural functions, more rapid reflex functions, lowered pain threshold, and sensitivity to stimuli. Balance is disturbed. The kidneys try to rebalance the increased alkalinity by excreting bicarbonates, and generalized imbalance occurs in the calcium and magnesium levels. This causes even more neurological mayhem, with cramps and spasms becoming more likely, accompanied by numbness, pins and needles, and possibly pain. These changes provide a superb environment for the evolution of myofascial trigger points, as they are known, to evolve in ischemic tissue where oxygen levels are low. All of this is pretty terrifying, and does little to calm the breathing rate!

Chronic fatigue and chronic pain problems (such as fibromyalgia) and a host of other health problems are characterized by just such breathing patterns. All of these symptoms are more likely in de-conditioned individuals because of the way their cells produce ATP (energy) in an anaerobic environment, creating acid wastes that further stimulate the breathing rate. Most can be eliminated or at the least improved, correcting the breathing pattern disorder.

From the *Naturopathy Digest*, January 2006, vol. I no. I, by Leon Chaitow, ND, DO, MRO. Dr. Chaitow is a practicing naturopath, osteopath, and acupuncturist in the UK, with over 30 years of clinical experience. He has written over 50 books and edits *The Journal of Bodywork and Movement Therapies*. He regularly lectures in the United States and Europe. He is Director of Research and Senior Therapeutic Advisor for the THERA (Therapy, Health Education and Research Association) Trust at one of the world's leading naturopathic clinics.

chronic hypocapnea should be tested for, using a capnometer, and more advanced corrective breathing work should be undertaken.

[See www.Breathing.com for more information.]

A related issue is people with chronically cold extremities, often medically diagnosed as Raynaud's Syndrome (disease or phenomenon). Our experience is that this again can be due to sympathetic dominance. The typical fight-or-flight response to stress and other factors is for the blood vessels to contract in the extremities while blood is redirected to the heart, brain, and larger muscle groups. People have come in for breathwork complaining, "I've always had cold hands and feet." After one session, through proper oxygenation and the calming effects of the parasympathetic shift, people will become warm and toasty in their extremities. I believe that at least one aspect of Reynaud's is a form of UDB (Undetected Dysfunctional Breathing) and yet, its symptoms will go away when the correct breathing pattern is introduced. Modern science refers to Raynaud's as "a disease that causes an interruption of blood flow to the fingers, toes, nose, and/or ears when a spasm occurs in the blood vessels of these areas. Spasms are caused by exposure to cold or emotional stress. Use of biofeedback, vasodilating medications, and other methods are helpful to some." [www.raynauds.org]

Sounds to me like hypocapnea, but it could have different ways of presenting. I would counsel breathworkers to treat it seriously, but to first see if it can be resolved simply by getting the client to breathe optimally rather than treating it as a disease that needs medication. It's interesting to note that the first use for hyperbaric oxygen chambers (immersion in high-compression 100% oxygen) in the 1940s was to stop the progression of gangrene. So we have a history of regressing gangrene and possibly Raynaud's through the application of oxygen.

Why not see what optimal breathing can do?

Denis Ouellette:

In the sidebar on the opposite page, Leon Chaitow is describing someone with chronic Undetected Dysfunctional Breathing (UDB), which can and should be addressed through corrective Optimal Breathing development techniques before such a person embarks upon breathwork. If such a "de-conditioned" person, as Chaitow describes, were encouraged to breathe in a pattern that was sympathetically activating (through high-chest or rapid breathing or forcing the air out on the exhale), then most likely tetany, anxiety, and discomfort would follow. Part of our work in Integral Breathwork and Optimal Breathing is to use a capnometer to monitor CO_2 levels in the exhale during breathwork. We expect the capnometer data will validate what our fieldwork already suggests, that the reactions described above can be exacerbated when sympathetic breathing is encouraged. The first half of our six-hour Integral Breathwork seminar involves optimal-breathing basics and coaching prior to breathwork.

In 25 years of breathwork, I've never seen a scenario as extreme as what Chaitow describes, but most breathworkers have seen tetany and people moving into sympathetic arousal, energy overload, and the release of trauma, which in itself, is more traumatic than necessary. We all want breathwork to be safe, gentle, and physiologically healing rather than jarring. Joy Manné, PhD, maintains that encouraging rapid, high-chest breathing during breathwork is tantamount to "raping the unconscious." [See Joy Manné's sidebar on page 111.]

The days of unschooled breathwork experimentation should be over. If breathwork therapy is to gain its place as the remarkably effective healing tool that it is, a solid understanding of breath physiology is needed, and the highest standards of safety and compassion for our clients must be maintained.

If you are a breathwork practitioner, I highly recommend you attend the Optimal Breathing School. Integral Breathwork incorporates some of the basic Optimal Breathing exercises as referred to in the Appendix. Establish a good parasympathetic breathing pattern and closely monitor it. Keep the attention on a full breath that starts in the diaphragm and encourage complete resting on the exhale (no excessive blowing out). When it appears that sympathetic arousal is approaching, encourage the client to slow their exhale down to help regain the O_2/CO_2 balance, and to reestablish a parasympathetic calm (note Tom Goode's recommendations in sidebar). Switching to nose breathing is advised if mouth breathing is being used. It's during these episodes when the greatest skills and experience of the facilitator are called upon. A primary goal of breathwork is to reestablish that wonderful well-being that comes when a person's fight-or-flight syndrome is resolved.

Our fieldwork indicates that when we teach and practice proper parasympathetic breathing before embarking on transformational breathwork, mild tetany is more apt to happen among the de-conditioned, i.e., those new to breathwork, those with UDB, those with energy-meridian blockages, those with a greater amount of stored trauma, or those who have become agitated and sympathetically activated during a session.

(Further chi-energy activation concepts are discussed by Daniel P. Reid and J. Michael Wood in the next article.)

When cramping and other uncomfortable symptoms occur during breathwork, Mike White says these clients need to "raise their energy thermostat," which is what Wilhelm Reich called, "increasing the energy building toleration." This must be achieved through gentle modulation. ▨

Michael Grant White, OBDMT, LMBT is located in Charlotte, North Carolina.
Phone: (866) 694-6425. E-mail: assist@breathing.com.

Mike is a health educator, personal growth mentor, breathing development specialist, author, public speaker, and vocalist who has successfully helped thousands transform their lives through correct breathing and nutrition. Mike is a somatic educator using the breath as a focal point for stress management, optimum health, emotional balance, self-expression, and personal power. He has combined key elements of Tibetan, Hatha, and Kundalini Yoga, Pranayama, Chi Kung (Qigong), Massage Therapy, Tai Chi, Karate, Reichian Therapy, Radiance Breathwork, Rebirthing, Meditation, Chanting, Toning, Operatic Training, Public Speaking, and Nutrition. He is a member of the American Holistic Medical Association, American Holistic Health Association, and a founding member of the Association of Humanistic Psychology Somatics Community. Testimonials from individuals he has worked with can be found at www.Breathing.com.

Mike's collaboration with Denis Ouellette has resulted in Integral Breathwork™ as introduced in Parts One and Three of this manual. Visit www.IntegralBreathwork.com.

Tetany: My Bottom Line

There's quite a bit on tetany in these pages—probably more than you will find anywhere. Are we belaboring it? Not when you consider how daunting it can feel for a first-time participant in breathwork. It's scary, uncomfortable, sometimes painful, and hard to get over. It occurs mainly in the hands and mouth areas. I agree with all the contributors here. Here are my tips, after facilitating many hundreds of sessions:

1) I've observed that tetany occurs most often in those of more slender build, with higher metabolisms, who tend to be more "tightly wound" in terms of how they are carrying stress.

2) I agree with Tom Goode (opposite) that it can be caused by breathing OUT too forcefully and thereby upsetting the delicate balance between oxygen and carbon-dioxide. I will usually get down on the floor next to the person's ear and guide them through slowing down their exhales by simply repeating: IN - 2 - 3 - 4... OUT - 2 - 3 - 4 - 5 - 6 - 7 - 8... This does work.

3) Lengthy explanations don't help the client. I always have them read the "What to Do • What to Expect" pages first (Chapter 10). Say something like: "You're blowing off a ton of stress. Relax on the exhale. There's a build-up—a traffic jam—at the exit points. Be patient. It will pass soon." It's helpful for them to know later that tetany lessens and stops after the first sessions.

4) Using the breathwork tools and techniques in this manual, I've found that difficult tetany occurs in 10-to-15% of first-time participants. Gentle massage and hand movements, as described here, can be relieving. The Zap-a-Kramp pillows (see Resources) contain common club moss, which is remarkably effective for the relieving of cramping. ▨

— Denis Ouellette • 2019

Avoiding Tetany Altogether

Tetany, or respiratory alkalosis, is caused by a pH imbalance when carbon dioxide leaves the body too rapidly. It occurs in breathing exercises when the exhale is forced or the breathing is focused in the chest, giving rise to sensations of tingling followed by muscle cramping. Tetany can be avoided altogether by allowing the breather to self-pace rather than breathe too quickly to a rhythm imposed by a drumbeat or evocative music.

In Full Wave Breathing¨, I have emphasized the 3:2 ratio of inhale to exhale because the longer inhales leave "tidal air" in the lungs. Usually this is sufficient to avoid tetany. I haven't encountered tetany in individual or group sessions for over ten years. Once each breather was allowed to be their own expert as to how fast to proceed, the problem of tetany simply disappeared. Should tetany arise, a quick solution to increase CO_2 and restore pH balance is to have the breather hold their breath.

Full Wave Breathing involves starting with the lower abdomen before moving the muscular action up into the solar plexus, the chest, the shoulders, and the back of the neck, in discrete movements. The emphasis throughout is upon slow, deep, full respiration and a complete softening of all the muscles on the exhale.

The full-wave movement includes all of the breathing muscles, including the scalene muscles at the back of the neck that hold the head upright. First, fill the lower lobes of the lungs, then the upper lobes. As the breath moves through the body, the shoulders lift but they do not shrug. Anyone visiting the web site will find full instructions.

The "slow and easy" prescription is also used to prevent symptoms arising from detoxification, which can produce flu-like aching and cold-like mucus production. Since most people are shallow breathers, it is normal for the body to start expelling toxins as the mind-body system is oxygenated.

Each of us is different and must find our own comfort level with our breathing exercises. Working with breathwork clients for over twenty-five years has taught me the value of trusting the integrity of each individual's mind-body system. When an unpleasant sensation is encountered for any reason during a breathwork session, it is a sign to back off, to ease the breathing depth and speed, and to find an accommodation that works for that person on that day. ▩

Tom Goode, ND, is the co-founder of the International Breath Institute; and the co-developer with Judith Kravitz of The Transformational Breath, which was later refined as Full Wave Breathing to be suitable for people of all levels of consciousness and physical condition. For more information and the free monthly e-zine, *Just Breathe!* visit www.InternationalBreathInstitute.com.

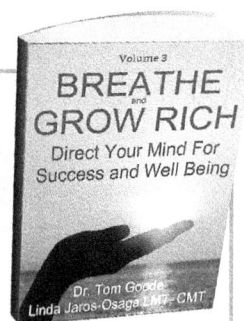

The Fire Hose

It's obvious to me that tetany is usually due to overbreathing, i.e., working too hard at breathing, pushing, blowing, or forcing too much on the exhale, focusing too much on breathing and not enough on relaxing. By overbreathing, people create unnecessary friction and stress in their system. When people relax on the exhale, they tend not to trigger tetany.

In the practice of *pranayama*, tetany is often explained in terms of *prana* and *apana*, two words for the same energy, but related to whether it is in-flowing (prana) or out-flowing (apana). If we take in more energy than we let out, or if we are slow to absorb or integrate it as it comes in, the energy simply piles up on us. So tetany, from this perspective, is a sign of imbalance or a lack of coordination, as when swallowing water when learning to swim or falling down when learning to walk. It's nothing to get upset about, to make rules or judgments against. It's not a reason to stop the learning or the healing process. My advice to people is, "It's just a feeling; try to relax and allow it to happen; just allow it roll through you."

One thing I'm certain of after working with thousands of people: tetany can occur with even slow or shallow breathing, with belly or chest breathing, and regardless of the inhale-to-exhale ratio. Emotional, psychological, and energetic factors can bring it on. The process of profound relaxation can trigger it. The intensity and duration of tetany seem more related to people's reaction to it. Resisting, fearing, judging, or suppressing it, or getting busy trying to make it go away, seem only to make it worse.

In general, I like to use the analogy of a fire hose when talking about tetany. A fire hose is soft and flexible like a body that is loose and relaxed. But when you connect the hose to a powerful water source, the hose appears to get stiff and hard when in fact it is still soft and flexible. The rigidity is due to the power of the water flowing through it. It's important not to confuse tension with power, intensity, and charge.

I tell people that tetany can be a sign of deep relaxation. It wouldn't occur unless something within them had opened enough to allow this powerful flow. I encourage people to trust this deeper part of themselves, to practice relaxing into the intense feelings, and to keep breathing in the direction of comfort and pleasure. Learning to relax and breathe through intense internal reactions can result in tremendous personal freedom. So we wouldn't do anything to deliberately intensify tetany, but we welcome the opportunity to breathe and relax into it.

When tetany occurs, I may coach people to use shallow breathing and encourage breath pauses, but I don't encourage breath holding. In general, when tetany distracts people from staying conscious with their breathing, I get them to focus more intently on relaxation and on trusting and allowing their physical, emotional, and psychological reactions to occur. ▪

Dan Brulé is a world-renowned healer and teacher and a founder of the worldwide spiritual breathing movement. Dan is one of the originators of breath therapy and was among the first group of internationally certified rebirthers. He is a leading member of Inspiration University, the International Rebirthers Association, and the International Breathwork Foundation. He is a master of *prana yoga* (the Hindu science of breath) and a Qigong master (Chinese medical breathing exercises). Visit www.BreathMastery.com.

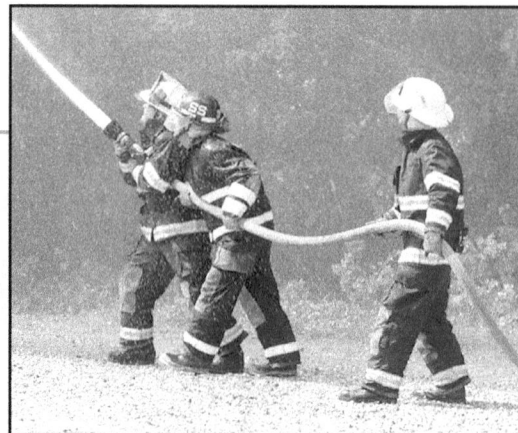

Working with Difficult Cases
Medications, Detox Symptoms & Chi Activation

Denis Ouellette, Michael Grant White & J. Michael Wood
with perspectives by Daniel P. Reid & Joy Manné

[EDITOR'S NOTE: This was a candid written interaction between myself (Denis), Michael Grant White (Mike), and J. Michael Wood (J. Michael). J. Michael is a Medical Qigong Practitioner; his comments and bio appear at the end of this article. This interaction is reprinted here because these are pertinent issues affecting all breathwork practitioners as we attempt to move from the traditional Western forms of medical practice, with their reliance on pharmaceutical drugs, to more natural methods of detoxing and healing.]

DENIS TO MIKE: Every once in a while, I'd say it's 2% of the time, someone will be quite headachy the next day after one of our breathwork seminars. Also, people who are on anti-depressants and other medications (which seems like a good percentage of the people nowadays) can have adverse symptoms and take longer to integrate their experience. In some cases, they may feel *worse* the next few days. I suspect that as oxygen moves in, the drugs and chemicals are being rejected by their cells, and the backlog of chemicals and toxins in their bodies are being dumped into the bloodstream for processing and eliminating. Other than the usual stuff about "healing crises and detox symptoms," anything you can add to this?

MIKE: Yes, it's a shame what the drug companies have given us and society to deal with.

DENIS: I want to be responsible in the book and mention somewhere that these things can happen. Often these people don't come back because they feel it's too much to go through. Those more understanding of natural healing may try it again. Detoxing from medications, especially antidepressants, is a really challenging issue. People can die from that. I don't want to take on the role of getting people off meds, or challenging doctors or psychiatrists. But it does come up, and it's very important to shift away from the meds mentality, but only for people who really want to do that.

MIKE: And some must have their MD guide them through that, and most MDs will not go there.

DENIS: Meds have their place and function, but they can also be like a steel cage. People can have their symptoms back off, but at a huge price to their health (producing a highly acidic body pH, side effects, etc.) and possibly at the expense of any real healing of the root cause of the issues. Here's a story: I had one guy come to me for a private breathwork session. He signed my release form, medical history and disclaimer, but he didn't tell me he was on meds for "hearing voices." He cried and got scared a lot in his session. It was like someone opened the door of his steel cage, but he was still staying inside, too scared to come out and walk through the door. A few days later, he called me back and said he had a good session, but he had started to hear the voices again so wished to discontinue the work.

MIKE: Yep. That is one thing that gets the psychotherapists up in arms about breathwork.

Chi Energy Activation

The act of breathing not only extracts chi from air, it also drives and distributes chi through the body's invisible network of energy channels, called "meridians." Meridians transport vital energy throughout the body and, when they get blocked, a condition called energy stagnation occurs.... Beginners should be prepared for several signs when commencing deep breathing regimens. There is a tendency to perspire and feel hot flashes in various parts of the body.... This is caused by heat released during cellular respiration and by the accelerated movement of vital energy throughout the meridian network....

Sometimes you'll feel "goose-bumps" or currents traveling up your spine, or down your arms and legs, or over the top of your head. This is chi moving through the meridians, propelled by the power of breath. The signs that disturb beginners most are occasional feelings of dizziness in the head, numbness or tingling in the extremities, and tremors in the muscles, but again, this is no cause for worry. It is the direct result of opening up long-neglected energy channels and pumping chi through them. As parts of the body chronically deprived of blood and energy are activated, they tend to tingle, just as when your foot "goes to sleep" and then you stand on it. With prolonged practice, all your channels will open up and energy will flow smoothly and evenly through the system, after which these tingly, dizzy feelings will disappear.

The Tao of Health, Sex and Longevity:
A Modern Practical Guide to the Ancient Way
Daniel P. Reid

DENIS: Breathwork *does* have the potential to heal serious mental and emotional issues, but these can be too big to take on, especially in a group-seminar setting; and often meds are already involved, so there's that dependency and the toxicity to deal with. Not everyone has the strength of Odysseus, who had himself strapped to the mast so he wouldn't be lured to destruction by the Sirens' voices. So it takes a very strong determination on the individual's part and a very solid support system in place (family, close daily contact with the therapist) to go through the detoxing.

MIKE: I agree, and how do you qualify such a person? When he told you he had no problems, he did not qualify himself honestly. That is what I mean about being careful with using hyperbole—making huge or grand statements about the healing potentials without adequate reality checks. Trouble is, the grand statements are often true. Time for some double-blind tests, don't you think?

DENIS: I'm working with a psychiatrist right now both with bodywork and breathwork. She described herself as "itchy and wobbly," said parts of it were painful, and was not fully integrated for a while after her breathwork session. She knows she needs to detox, get off anti-depressants, and get her life back in balance from over-work, etc. Then she'll be looking for some new tools to share with her clients. She knows that her profession (in her own words) is "imploding" because of the strangle-hold of drugs. She was not at ease with the group session, perhaps due to the psychiatrist-client format of her own practice, and is now somewhat "ambivalent" about continuing with the work.

MIKE: Talk to J. Michael Wood, Optimal Breathing School core faculty member, who is a Medical Qigong Master. He works in a psychiatrist's office in Nashville. Call him and talk to him about all this. He is expecting your call.

DENIS: I believe that the conditions associated with overactive sympathetic tone (see *Our Nervous Systems* in Appendix) will lessen as breathing development and breathwork are engaged in. When people I'm working with are showing improvement in their conditions and ask me for a solution to getting off meds, I ask them to work with their doctors and consider taking a razor blade to shave off a small amount dosage each day. Then over many days, they will have safely shaved it all away.

DENIS TO J. MICHAEL: Any comments on this, J. Michael? Also, it would be great if you could share your expertise regarding the issue of how psychologists, psychiatrists, massage therapists, etc., take on the energy of their clients—how this energy transference is part of what they're dealing with when they start their own breathwork and healing work—and any specific ways you deal with this overloaded state. Thanks.

J. MICHAEL: Hi, Denis. You indicated that on occasion after a session of breathwork, some participants had a reaction of "wobbly, itchy and/or headachy." From a standpoint of Chinese Medicine, it might be observed as follows:

Wobbly: The unsteady feeling is generally a sign the person has become ungrounded. One breathing technique that has been successful for me is to have them focus on inhaling and exhaling through their heels. After three or four breaths like this, direct them to imagine their heels are in the center of the earth and to continue to imagine breathing through the heels.

Itchy: This generally indicates that the meridian system is opening (or reopening), and the *chi* energy is becoming unblocked. Additionally, this can show that the parasympathetic response has been triggered and the peripheral artery system has begun to dilate.

In both of these and most cases of this nature, the breathing pattern I would recommend would be a purging breath where the exhale should be longer than the inhale by at least half, i.e., inhale on a four-count and exhale on a six-count, and complete the exhale with "la-la-la-la..." to extend the excursion of the diaphragm and to help trigger the parasympathetic or relaxation response.

Headachy: The headaches are many times one or both of the following:

1. Detoxing that drains and overloads the lymph system. This will be evidenced by swelling and tenderness in the glands just below the collarbones (approximately in line with the sides of the neck). If this is evidenced, have them massage the glands deeply and then massage the trigger point in the web between the thumb and forefinger on each hand.

2. The cathartic effect of the breathwork can cause toxic issues to surface, especially repressed anger. This can cause a toxic overload from the liver, which is expressed through the gall bladder meridians on the head. A simple way to try to unblock the meridians is to massage the trigger points on the back approximately opposite the lymph glands.

These techniques have consistently been helpful in the adjunctive therapy I provide to patients referred by a psychiatrist. I hope this will be of help as you go forward in dealing with the more difficult cases.

Regarding the picking up of energy, I have noticed that psychiatrists, psychologists, and bodyworkers in general all are vulnerable to ingesting the toxic energy of the people they treat. One patient I treated was a masters' level nurse who worked in the intensive care unit treating thoracic postoperative patients. She suffered from constant migraines and seizures (both cataleptic and epileptic). As I questioned her about her job prior to her total disability, she said when a patient went into crisis they would "bust open the chest," and attempt to save them. Imagine standing over the open chest of a patient *in extremis* and inhaling the toxic energy. It was little wonder that she was disabled.

Psychiatrists and psychologists are also inhaling the toxic energy of their disturbed patients one after another, all day long. Most of the time, they are running behind and are not eating properly, which creates weakness in their energy field. None of the ones I personally have seen have proper breathing mechanics, and I believe this is amping up the stress at an unbelievable rate. It is little wonder that cathartic breathwork might put them in distress as they begin to shed the toxic energy.

My first line of defense for this situation is to teach them a safe place with the breath, using the complete exhale with "la-la-la-la" to trigger the parasympathetic response. I have them breathe in and out through the heels, and then have them imagine the heels are deeply rooted in the earth.

I have used these techniques in real-world situations with this type of professional, and have been able to pull them out of their agitated states. I hope this will be of value to the ones that your work is reaching.

J. Michael Wood, PBMC, OBDS, MMQ lives in Nashville, TN. Phone: (615) 366-8940. E-mail: jmw@breathing.com. Visit www.QigongMedicine.com.

Michael has been practicing alternative health modalities for 38 years. During the last 7 years, he has trained in breathwork with Drs. Gay and Kathlyn Hendricks of the Hendricks Institute, and with Michael Grant White. He is certified as a Professional Breath and Movement Coach with Hendricks, and as an Optimal Breathing Development Specialist with White. In addition, he received a Masters of Medical Qigong from the International Institute of Medical Qigong (IIMQ), and has taken advanced Medical Qigong training in cancer therapy from Dr. Jerry Alan Johnson, Dean of the IIMQ. J. Michael has been accepted by the AOBTA as a Certified Practitioner in Medical Qigong, is in private practice with Medical Qigong, and provides adjunctive therapy in breathwork at the Center for Integrated Health in Nashville.

Michael is serving as core faculty member of the Optimal Breathing School and Director of the Middle Tennessee Branch of the International Institute of Medical Qigong, where he is presently teaching the 200-hour course for certification as a Medical Qigong Practitioner.

Tip for Breathwork Facilitators:
THE BIG RED FLASHING NEON ARROW!

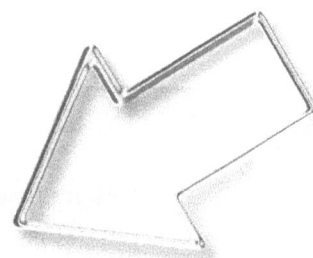

When assisting someone through their breathwork, always pay attention to the subtle (and sometimes not so subtle) cues, movements, and statements they make. Keep in mind that everything in their world is amplified right now. Their sensitivities are acute. Always respond in some helpful but gentle way to every little thing they show or tell you. Treat every little sign as if it is a large, flashing neon arrow, telling you something about what they need. If they lick their lips, dry from so much mouth breathing, ask them if you can drop a sip of water into their mouth. They may say, "My chest feels so tight!" This may be a very old blockage of energy that's ready to release. Sometimes verbal encouragement works well. "It's OK to release that now," or "Let's place our hands there and breathe into that area." Light touch or massage may be appropriate, with permission. If you have crystals handy, and they're into that, ask them what they want, "I have pink, clear or green..." and where to place it. They will know intuitively. As spoken of in Part Two, crystals do absorb negative energies and transmit helpful earth energy.

—*Editor*

Nothing as Powerful as Gentleness

CONSCIOUS
BREATHING:
*How Shamanic Breathwork
Can Transform Your Life*

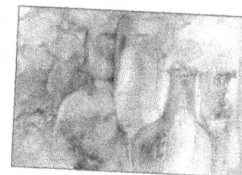

Joy Manné
Author of Soul Therapy

Dear Denis,

I had a chance to read this article tonight and found it interesting. I do not work with people on any form of drugs or medications, so I have no personal experience to contribute there.

However, if you read the section on "Unloading" in my book, *Conscious Breathing,* you will have the essence of my approach. If someone simply has their attention on their breathing, and this person is sitting up and not lying down—so there is no changing or interfering with the breathing rhythm by the facilitator, no imposition of connected breathing or anything else, where the technique is just letting the body breathe in its own rhythm—then something will come up. It could be something traumatic, something that distresses the person, but it will be something manageable. It will not overwhelm the client. I think any other kind of breathing with people who are so traumatized that they are on medication will be far too much and will retraumatize them.

What I see again and again is that in all personal and spiritual development (and therapy), slow is considered fast if the "slow" is grounded and aimed towards building a good foundation. "Fast" is destabilizing and therefore ends up slowing or stopping the person's progress. Just teaching a person abdominal breathing—the first thing I do with all clients, individually and in groups— is already a revelation for most people. You can read how I discovered this in *Soul Therapy.*

I do have clients lying down for a transformational breathing session, but the sitting-up breathing is equally transformational. All the altered states read about can happen during a sitting-up session. If the wisdom of the body is accessed, and the body is allowed to breathe at its own rhythm, experiences that can be integrated and that do not retraumatize will come up. Everything that is best about breathwork will happen. The body, and the Soul, will guide the process. Especially for those who have been traumatized, nothing is as powerful as gentleness. That is what I wrote in my breathwork novel, which I am preparing for publication.

I hope that's useful.

Cordially,

Joy

Joy Manné, Ph.D., author of *Soul Therapy*; and *Conscious Breathing: How Shamanic Breathing Can Transform Your Life.* Editor of *The Healing Breath: A Journal of Breathwork Practice, Psychology and Spirituality.* Visit www.HealingBreathJournal.org and www.i-Breathe.com.

Sound, Intention & Genetic Healing

Sol Luckman

In an intriguing section of a fascinating book entitled *The Cosmic Serpent: DNA and the Origins of Knowledge*, French anthropologist Jeremy Narby includes snippets from his personal journals from his time spent studying the healing practices of Amazonian medicine men. One entry is of particular interest on the popular subject of genetic healing.

"According to shamans of the entire world," writes Dr. Narby, communication with healing spirits is established "via music. For [shamans] it is almost inconceivable to enter the world of spirits and remain silent. Angelica Gebhart Sayer discusses the visual music projected by the spirits in front of the shaman's eyes. It is made up of three-dimensional images that coalesce into sound, and that the shaman imitates by emitting corresponding melodies." In a provocative footnote to himself, Narby adds, "I should check whether DNA emits sound or not."

One school of thought insists that humans are actually made of sound and that DNA itself may be a form of sound. Drawing on meticulously documented research, Harvard-trained Leonard Horowitz explains that DNA emits and receives both phonons and photons, or electromagnetic waves of sound and light. In the 1990s, according to Dr. Horowitz, "three Nobel laureates in medicine advanced research that revealed the primary function of DNA lies not in protein synthesis...but in the realm of bio-acoustic and bioelectric signaling." In recent years a new artistic field called DNA music has even begun to flourish. It therefore seems appropriate, at the very least, to compare DNA to a keyboard with a number of keys that produce the music of life.

But what if on some level we are made of sound? What if in the beginning was the Word? What if the music of the spheres is no myth? What if we ourselves are a harmonic conver-

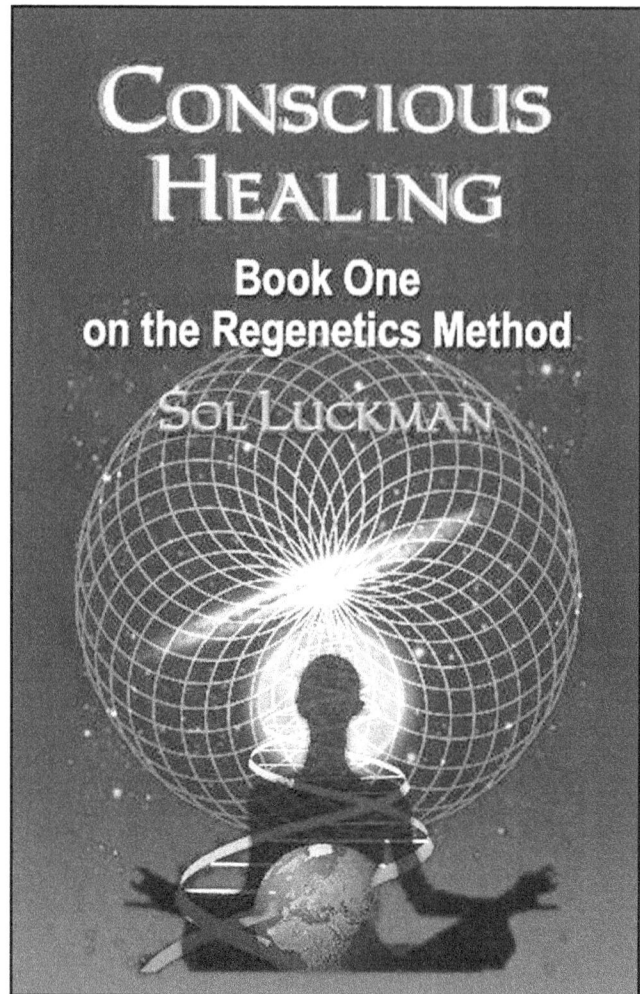

gence? What if the holographic grid of our being is a linguistic and musical interface between higher-dimensional light, which might be considered a form of divine thought or intention, and sound in higher-dimensional octaves? After all, String theory posits the existence of many different, theoretically accessible dimensions that appear notationally linked much like strings on a guitar.

Narby repeatedly makes the point that shamans use sound because this allows them to transform some aspect of the genetic code. If DNA is indeed a text, a keyboard, a musical score; if it is true that this score can be rewritten so that it plays a new type of music; and if we live not just in a holographic but in a harmonic universe, then it seems plausible that our bioenergy fields are at least in part composed of higher-dimensional sound.

When my partner Leigh and I began developing a method of DNA activation called Regenetics, we discovered through kinesiology (muscle testing) that each of the body's auric or electromagnetic fields corresponds not just to a chakra but to a third-dimensional sound octave. Energetically, our research indicates that humans are built of a vertical series of light-processing chakras interfacing with concentric electromagnetic fields (which are sonic in nature) to form the three-dimensional holographic matrix that produces our physical body.

At the genetic level, sound gives rise to light. In a paper entitled "A Holographic Concept of Reality" appearing in *Psychoenergetic Systems* in 1975, a team of researchers headlined by Richard Alan Miller first outlined a compelling model of "ener-genetic" expression resulting in "precipitated reality": "Superposed coherent waves of different types in the cells interact to form diffraction patterns, firstly in the acoustic [sound] domain, secondly in the electromagnetic [light] domain." This leads to the manifestation of physical form as a "quantum hologram—a translation between acoustical and optical holograms." Significantly, this sound-light translation mechanism that creates the somatic experience of reality functions in the genome.

This is not the place to provide a full treatment of the science of quantum bioholography. Rather, I wish to emphasize that according to this model that is attracting many proponents as more and more of its precepts are confirmed, it is becoming apparent that DNA directs cellular metabolism and replication not just biochemically but electromagnetically through a chromosomal mechanism that translates sound into light waves, and vice versa. Sound and light, or phonons and photons, establish a sophisticated communication network throughout the physical organism that extends into the bioenergy fields and back to the cellular and subcellular levels.

Recalling Edgar Cayce's prediction that "sound would be the medicine of the future," Jonathan Goldman, in *Healing Sounds: The Power of Harmonics,* coined the following inspirational formula: sound + intention = healing. If we define intention as a form of conscious light energy roughly equivalent to thought, an idea consistent with many shamanic traditions such as that of the Toltecs of Mesoamerica, we can translate Goldman's formula as:

SOUND + LIGHT = HEALING.

Recently, the ability of sound and light to heal DNA was scientifically documented by a Russian research team of geneticists and linguists. Russian linguists discovered that the genetic code, especially in the so-called junk portion, follows regular grammar and usage rules virtually identical to those of human languages. This invalidates many modern linguistic theories by proving that language did not appear randomly but reflects humanity's shared genetics. In *The God Code,* bestselling author Gregg Braden further demonstrates that the ancient four-letter Hebrew name for God (YHVH, *Yod Hey Vav Hey*) is actually code for DNA based on the latter's chemical composition of nitrogen, oxygen, hydrogen, and carbon. This assertion, with its vast implications relative to DNA's universal role as a divine language spoken through the body, has been peer-reviewed and accepted by many scholars of Hebrew.

Fritz Albert Popp's Nobel Prize-winning research establishes that every cell in the body receives, stores and emits coherent light in the form of biophotons. In tandem with biophonons, biophotons maintain electromagnetic frequency patterns in all living organisms. ▪

What if on some level we are made of sound? What if in the beginning was the Word? What if the music of the spheres is no myth? What if we ourselves are a harmonic convergence? What if the holographic grid of our being is a linguistic and musical interface between higher-dimensional light, which might be considered a form of divine thought or intention, and sound in higher-dimensional octaves?

In the words of Dr. Stephen Lindsteadt, this matrix that is produced and sustained by frequency oscillations "provides the energetic switch-boarding behind every cellular function, including DNA/RNA messaging. Cell membranes scan and convert signals into electromagnetic events as proteins in the cell's bi-layer change shape to vibrations of specific resonant frequencies." Emphasizing that every "biochemical reaction is preceded by an electromagnetic signal," Lindsteadt concludes, "Cells communicate both electromagnetically and chemically and create biochemical pathways that interconnect all functions of the body."

> When we use our minds to think, we are creating movements of electrical impulses in the brain, and when any electrical energy moves, torsion waves are also created.
>
> —David Wilcock
>
> This spiraling 'torsion' energy could actually be the substance of our human souls, and is therefore the precursor to the DNA molecule.... It already exists in the fabric of space and time before any physical life emerges.
>
> —Wynn Free

Russian scientists Peter Gariaev and Vladimir Poponin have also explored DNA's extraordinary electromagnetic properties. Their research shows that DNA has a special ability to attract photons, causing the latter to spiral along the helix-shaped DNA molecule instead of proceeding along a linear path. In other words, DNA has the amazing ability—unlike any other molecule known to exist—to bend or weave light around itself.

In addition, it appears that a previously undetected form of intelligent light or intention energy (emanating from higher dimensions and distinguishable from both gravity and electromagnetic radiation), which Dr. Eli Cartan first termed "torsion" in 1913, after its twisting movement through the fabric of space-time, gives rise to DNA. Many decades later, the concept of torsion energy was still alive and well enough to inspire an entire generation of Russian scientists, who authored thousands of papers on the subject in the 1990s alone. "A unified subliminal field of potentially universal consciousness apparently exists," writes Horowitz on the subject of the Russian studies, "and may be explained as emerging from a previously overlooked physical vacuum."

The ancient Greeks were well aware of this potent energy, calling it *aether* and understanding that it is directly responsible for universal manifestation. In the 1950s, Russian scientist Nicolai Kozyrev conclusively proved the existence of this life-giving subspace energy, demonstrating that, like time, it flows in a sacred geometric spiral that has been called *phi*, the Golden Mean, and the Fibonacci sequence. In the face of overwhelming evidence of its existence, modern scientists are returning to the notion of *aether* using such phrases as "zero point energy" and "vacuum potential." Recently, physicists Richard Feynman and John Wheeler went so far as to calculate that the amount of torsion energy contained inside a light bulb could literally bring the world's oceans to a boil!

This breakthrough research in the temporal physics of subspace establishes that torsion energy permeates the entire multidimensional galaxy and, not only is responsive to, but may actually be consciousness creatively experiencing itself in time. "To put it as bluntly as possible," writes renowned psychic and gifted scientific researcher David Wilcock, "you cannot separate consciousness and torsion waves—they are the same thing.

When we use our minds to think, we are creating movements of electrical impulses in the brain, and when any electrical energy moves, torsion waves are also created."

According to the Russian findings, notes author Wynn Free, "this spiraling 'torsion' energy could actually be the substance of our human souls, and is therefore the precursor to the DNA molecule....It already exists in the fabric of space and time before any physical life emerges." Elsewhere, Free remarks of transposons that these tiny segments of DNA can travel along the genome activating different parts of it when prompted by consciousness. In keeping with Dr. Gariaev's "Wave-based Genome" theory, Free concludes that DNA functions "somewhat like a computer chip, with different sections that can either be 'on' or 'off.'" Thus we can easily imagine how the torsion waves of human consciousness could program, or reprogram, DNA's binary code.

Similarly, the Gariaev group demonstrated that chromosomes function much like (re)programmable holographic biocomputers employing DNA's own electromagnetic radiation. Their research strongly suggests that human DNA is literally a genetic "text"—that chromosomes both produce and receive the information contained in these texts in order to encode and decode them, respectively—and that chromosomes assemble themselves into a holographic grating or lattice

designed to generate and interpret highly stable spiral standing waves of sound and light that direct all biological functions. In other words, explain longtime genetics researchers Iona.

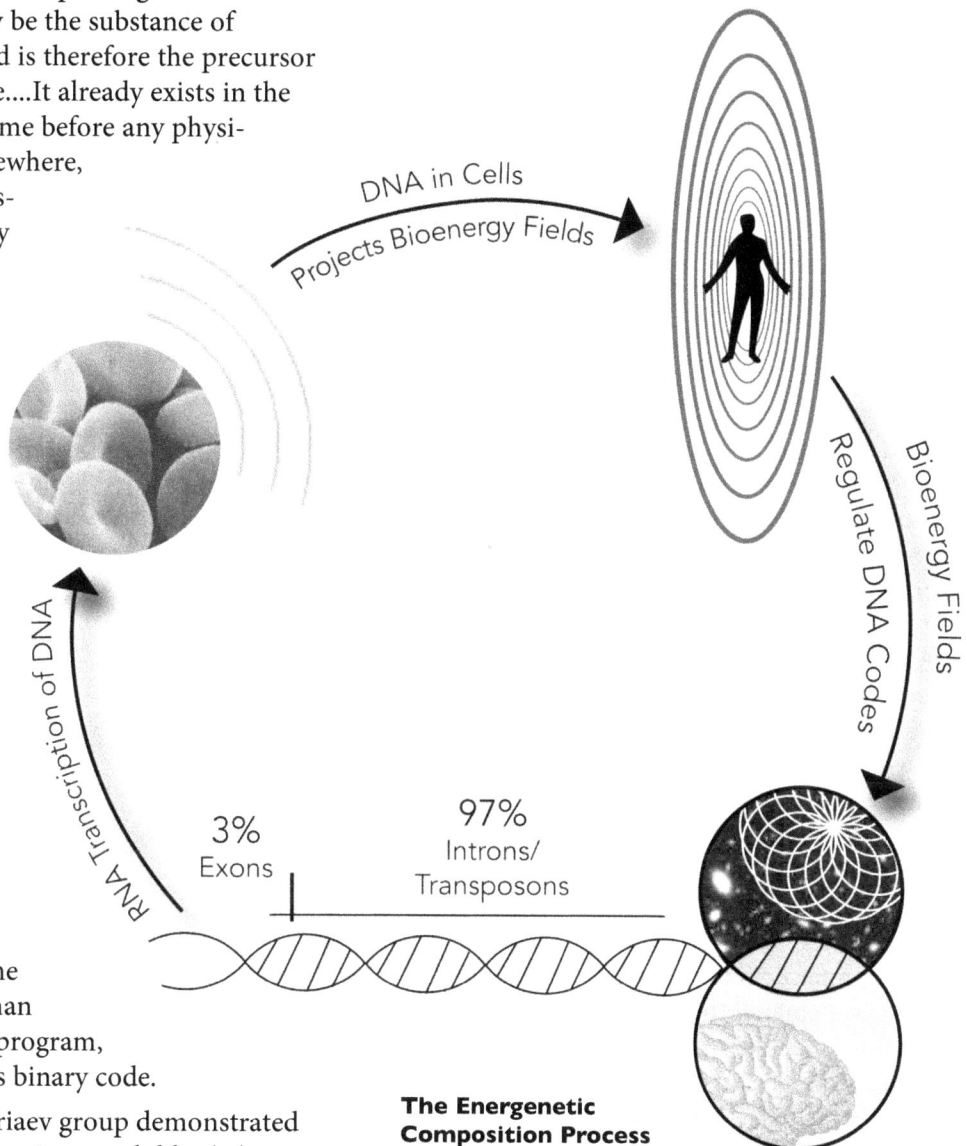

DNA in Cells
Projects Bioenergy Fields

Bioenergy Fields
Regulate DNA Codes

RNA Transcription of DNA

3%
Exons

97%
Introns/
Transposons

The Energenetic Composition Process
from *Conscious Healing: Book One on the Regenetics Method.* The above diagram illustrates how cell building is both genetic, involving RNA transcription of DNA codes to create cells, and energetic, dependent on the interface between the electromagnetic fields and the supposedly unused 97% of the DNA molecule, or Potential DNA, for regulation of cellular composition. This diagram also shows how potential DNA's transposons can be directly prompted to modify cellular replication by consciousness, both internal (personal) and external (universal).

Miller and Richard Alan Miller in a superb article based partly on Gariaev's findings entitled, "From Helix to Hologram," DNA's "code is transformed into physical matter, guided by light and sound signals."

Decades of research by Dr. Kikuo Chishima, a Japanese scientist, suggest that red blood cells are formed not in bone marrow, as is commonly believed, but in the intestinal villi. Red blood cells appear to be: 1) guided by systemic frequency oscillations manifesting in the bioenergy blueprint and 2) capable of synthesizing DNA in order to differentiate into specific types of cells, which then migrate via the 90,000-mile-long capillary system to wherever they are needed. Writes Lindsteadt, "This open-ended system that connects to the lymphatic system, the meridian system and the connective tissue provides communication pathways for the flow of information and cellular instructions from the electromagnetic energy matrix."

One revolutionary corollary (to many) of this research is that, to activate DNA and stimulate healing on the cellular level, one can simply use our species' supreme expression of creative consciousness: words. While Western researchers clumsily cut and splice genes, Gariaev's team developed sophisticated devices capable of influencing cellular metabolism through sound and light waves keyed to human language frequencies. Using this method, Gariaev proved that chromo-

somes damaged by X-rays, for instance, can be repaired. Moreover, this was accomplished noninvasively by simply applying vibration and language, or sound combined with intention, or words, to DNA.

According to Iona Miller and Richard Miller, "Life is fundamentally electromagnetic rather than chemical, the DNA blueprint functioning as a biohologram which serves as a guiding matrix for organizing physical form." Arguably the most far-reaching implication of the research cited in this article is that DNA can be activated through conscious linguistic expression (somewhat like an antenna) to reset the bioenergy fields, which in turn (like orbiting communication satellites) can transmit radio and light signals to restore the proper cellular structure and functioning of the human body.

> One revolutionary corollary…of this research is that, to activate DNA and stimulate healing on the cellular level, one can simply use our species' supreme expression of creative consciousness: words…. Gariaev's team developed sophisticated devices capable of influencing cellular metabolism through sound and light waves keyed to human language frequencies…prov[ing] that chromosomes damaged by X-rays, for instance, can be repaired. Moreover, this was accomplished noninvasively by simply applying vibration and language, or sound, combined with intention, or words, to DNA.

Sol Luckman is editor of *DNA Monthly* and cofounder of the Phoenix Center for Regenetics, offering cutting-edge educational services and materials designed to activate unity consciousness and actualize human potential. The developers of the Regenetics Method are educators and ordained ministers, not medical doctors, and do not purport to diagnose or treat illness. The preceding article is adapted from *Conscious Healing: Book One on the Regenetics Method*, by Sol Luckman. For information visit www.phoenixregenetics.org.

The naturally occurring electric fields that surround us and penetrate us are understood and utilized by many of today's complementary and alternative health practitioners. These forces play a vital role in keeping our bodies healthy. Hundreds of books have discussed the eastern interpretations of this energy. The intent of this article is to provide Western scientific theoretical support for how complementary and alternative medicine (CAM) approaches work. We will discuss acupuncture, breathwork, bodywork, and energy work (Therapeutic Touch, Reiki, etc.), Tai Chi, Qigong, feng shui, radon mines, natural-spring spas, mountain and seaside dwelling, and how our Nyvatex Health-Mat™ fits with CAM approaches.

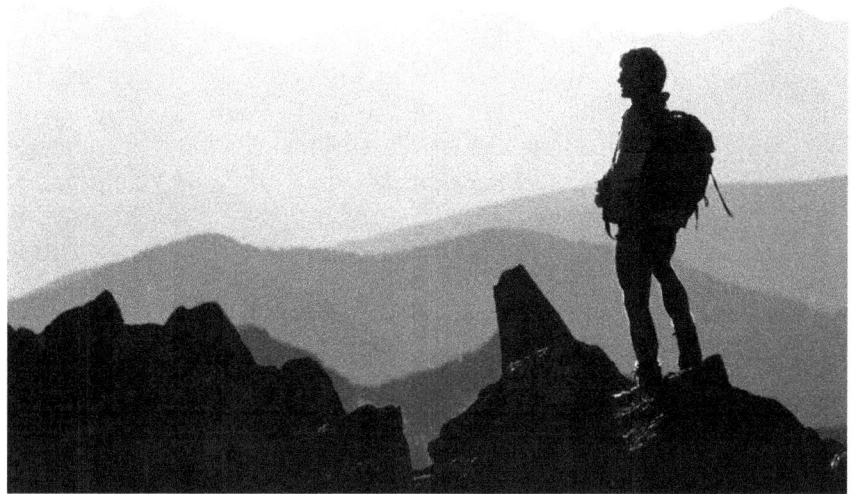

The Earth's & Our Body's Health-Enhancing Electric Fields

John C. Ledbetter

Underlying all these methods is the manipulation and application of nature's electric fields. How well these methods work is dependent upon whether they afford the body improved access to (or how well they boost) these internal and external electric fields. Let's start with how the earth's external fields affect the body, and then show how the body's internal fields are essential for healthy living, for healing, and for supporting healthy aging.

Living higher in altitude means living longer and healthier. There are a vast number of anecdotal stories of healthy people who spent their lives in mountains. A study published in the April, 2005, issue of The Journal of Epidemiology and Community Health reveals that residents of a Greek village at 3,100 feet lived longer and had less heart disease compared to residents of two similar villages located at sea level. The earth's atmospheric electric field increases approximately 100 volts for every meter one goes up in altitude towards the ionosphere. Thus 3,100 feet of altitude translates to approximately 100,000 more

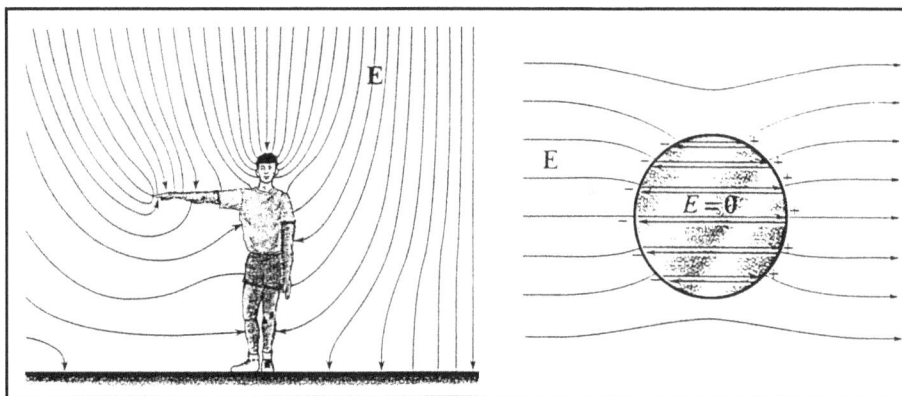

Figure A. Man standing outside in the earth's atmospheric electric field. Electric field lines are always perpendicular at the point of contact with an electrical conductor, of which the human body is a good one. If electric fields were in the visible range, you would see a rainbow-colored forest of electric field lines shooting out of the ground everywhere, stretching up to the ionosphere. All living things have evolved and developed within this field, and we need it every day for good health. A zero electric field is created inside metal cars or trucks, trains and planes, aluminum-sided homes, etc. (represented by the circle). The atmospheric electric field cannot reach the occupants at full strength. Without this field effect, your body gets "sick" because it does not have access to the life-force energy it needs to efficiently heal itself or maintain health.

volts of electric-field intensity than what exists at sea level. The villagers don't feel this, as there are little-to-no amperes (electrical current) involved, but the voltage is there nonetheless.

Dr. Nikos Baibas, of the Department of Hygiene and Epidemiology at the University of Athens, was the main author on this study that examined 1,198 village residents. The three villages are about 125 miles from Athens. Mortality from heart disease in the mountain village was 54% lower for women and 61% lower for men, even though the mountain residents on average had higher blood pressure and higher total cholesterol and triglycerides than those in the two low-lying villages. The villagers were of the same genetic background, and about the same diet and lifestyle. The only difference was the altitude.

Death rates from all other causes were also lower in the mountains. In all three villages, the principal occupations were farming and animal breeding, and women were mainly responsible for household activities. The men were outside more than the women, and I interpret this to be why heart disease was lower for the men. The simple reason was the men's more-frequent outdoor immersion in the earth's atmospheric electrical field. Could this explain why people love going to the mountains and why many health rehabilitation resorts are located in the mountains?

For many years, I researched over 600 of the earth's famous healing sites and visited quite a few, including mineral springs, health spas, American Indian medicine circles, mountaintop

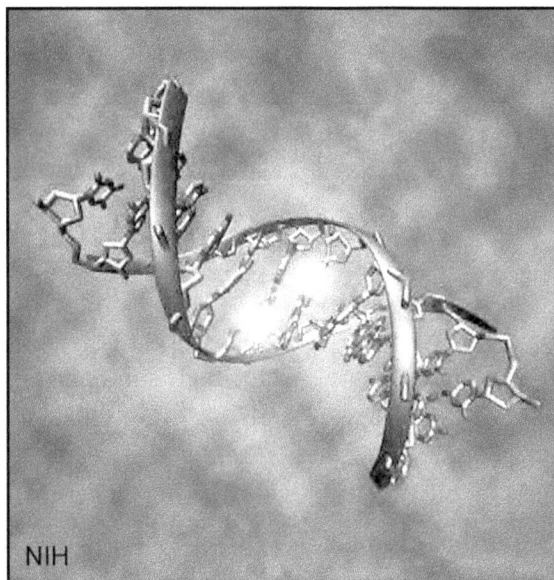

Figure B. THE SPARK OF HEALTHY LIFE. Note flashes of light in the center. DNA shown repairing itself using natural electric fields as their energy source, from inside and outside the body. Mutated malformed DNA that cannot repair itself can cause disease. In a healthy body these are destroyed by a robust immune system. Only healthy DNA, spontaneously self-repaired as necessary, produces healthy life. More info at www.DNArenew.com.

retreats, radon mines, and more, seeking a common scientific explanation for their health-enhancing effects. I found that each of these locations included a physical phenomenon that increased the electric-field energy available to visitors. This is my analysis as to how these healing sites work for healing and health maintenance.

1. Most mountains have stronger electric fields because they are nearer to the earth's ionosphere. Cosmic rays tend to ionize the air more where the air is thinner, making it more electrically conductive, thereby increasing the electric-field transfer to the body. Radioactive decay from metamorphosed rock also ionizes the air.

2. Many healing sites at all elevations have more active gamma radiation from radioactive decay of concentrations of thorium. This small increase in gamma-ray radiation ionizes the air, making it more electrically conductive. This too enables greater electric-field charge to the body.

3. Mine-shaft sites containing radon are considered therapeutic for a wide range of ailments. The radon from radioactive decay also ionizes the air, enabling electric-field transfer to the body, both externally through the skin and internally through inhalation.

4. Salty seashore air is more electrically conductive and thereby increases electric-field contact transfer to the body, both internally and externally. (Offshore breezes blowing onto Caribbean islands are called "doctor winds" by natives.)

My research on healing sites led me to the development of the patented Nyvatex Health-Mat, a simple device that would create and amplify the atmospheric electric field and be available to everyone wherever they were on the planet. The user could enjoy the benefits daily with no change in routine or lengthy visits to healing sites. My design criteria included ease of use, simplicity, and affordability. I was successful with the health-mat, as thousands of happy users have reported. (See Figure A for an illustration of atmospheric electric fields and an explanation of how modern life limits our access to them.)

Now let's examine the body's use of internally generated electric fields. It is well accepted that all degenerative and chronic diseases are a result of malfunctioning DNA. In a healthy-functioning body, the DNA resident within each cell is constantly repairing itself so as to maintain its function as the basis for life. When DNA cannot repair or renew itself, and the immune system is not sufficiently robust to eliminate the mutated DNA, disease begins to develop. Twenty-five years may transpire between the initial survival of malfunctioning DNA and the appearance of a diagnosable disease. That's why most chronic diseases (as well as cancer) show up in middle age or older (see Figure B).

Almost as soon as the structure of DNA was decoded, biochemists began speculating that the double helix might do more than just store information. Its chemical structure suggested it could conduct electricity just like copper wire. In living cells, DNA soaks up an electric charge and transports it over long distances to power spontaneous repair. In living cells DNA is bundled up with proteins and coiled into impenetrable helices. The ability of the double helix to conduct electricity plays a fundamental role in the front line of

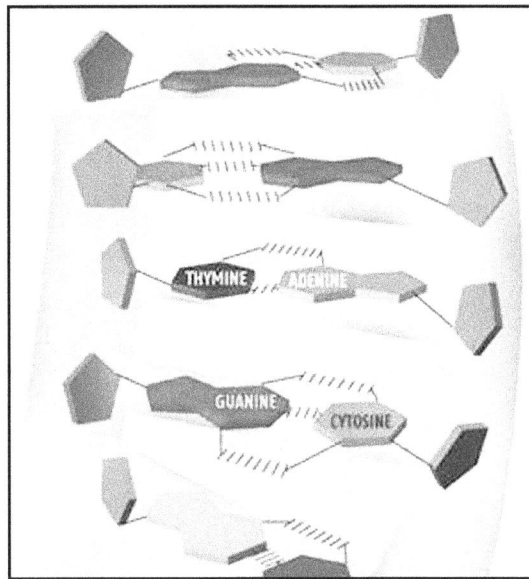

Figure C. Tight packing of DNA bases enables electric charge conduction. The natural electric potential of each base pair depends on electric charge differentials (REDOX potentials). DNA is tightly packed—an average DNA strand unfolds to about six feet.

defense against mutations. The tight stacking of bases allows a charge to be conducted along the helix (see Figure C). By externally boosting the electric field, DNA is helped to repair itself. Within my theory, this is also how CAM approaches work to provide an electric field boost to DNA:

1. Acupuncture employs needles. These needles serve as antennae concentrating the atmospheric electric field at specific points along the energy channels in the body (meridians), much like lightning rods provide the preferred path for lightning. The sharp tip of the needles ionize nearby air molecules by cold emission, making them more electrically conductive. Lightning is a concentration of the earth's atmospheric electric field. Feng shui is the oriental practice of directing these same electric fields to best availability in dwellings.

2. Tai Chi, Qigong and yoga postures allow the body to act as a free-form antenna. While most Americans perform these indoors on insulating surfaces, they work best outdoors and while barefoot or wearing thin slippers to establish ground contact (just as a lightning rod is grounded).

3. Therapeutic Touch, Reiki, and other bodywork modalities take advantage of the practitioners' ability to concentrate and send electric fields through their hands. The electric fields are sourced externally from the earth, and internally from the cells' self-generated electric fields.

4. Breathwork increases the intake of negatively charged ions from the air, which creates energy flow along the meridians. Breathing in naturally occurring negative ions aids

electric-field conductivity inside the lungs and throughout the body. Properly controlled breathing will efficiently oxygenate the blood, dispelling the clustering of blood cells, freeing each cell to independently establish healthy, self-generated, natural electric fields as nature intended for internal cellular health. The body discards about 200 million used red blood cells daily. Efficient intake of ionized air and oxygen is essential for the full functioning of 200 million replacement red blood cells, as well as healthy maintenance of the existing ones.

5. The Nyvatex Health-Mat employs a phenomenon called "triboelectrification," a process of electrical charge separation that involves the rubbing together (friction) of dissimilar material surfaces, to create, capture, amplify and boost an equivalent to the earth's electric field under and around the user. The mat also slightly ionizes nearby air. You just sleep or sit on it. [See ad in Resources or visit www.health-mat.com.]

There are 100 trillion cells in the human body. Nature has provided each cell with the ability to generate its own electric field for life, health and spontaneous DNA self-healing and self-repair. This is accomplished through a process known as the "sodium-potassium pump" (see Figure D).

Internally generated electric fields are an inevitable product of biological systems. Cell membranes and epithelia (flat sheets of cells such as the outer layer of your skin and the lining of your gut) routinely pump ions from one side to the other, creating gradients in electrical potential. This makes them resemble charged batteries, with an excess of negative ions on one side and positive ions on the other. All it takes for current to flow is for a channel to open up, linking the two sides. Where there is a current flowing, an electric field inevitably follows.

Researchers have measured naturally occurring electric fields in organisms ranging from microbes to humans. The strength of the fields is typically between 10 and 100 millivolts per millimeter, but can sometimes reach up to 1600 millivolts per millimeter. Many of those researchers believe that full understanding of these electric fields and their effects will lead to great medical advances. "I think understanding the bioelectrical energies involved in life processes will open up possibilities as great, or greater, than those resulting from the recent revolutions in molecular genetics [The Human Genome Project]," says Michael Levin, of the Forsyth Institute in Boston, Massachusetts.

Those successfully practicing CAM methods are already showing these "great possibilities" to be true in their daily applications. Through the understanding of electric-field healing and health maintenance theory, conventional and CAM methods can meet and jointly provide better

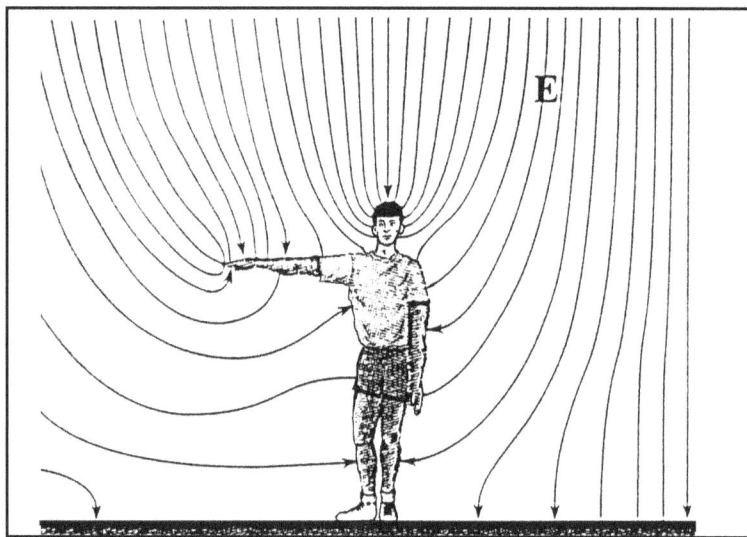

Figure D. Schematic of Sodium (Na) and Potassium (K) charge differentials which create a naturally occurring electric-battery pump, and from which each cell generates its own power for healing, health and life—the original renewable energy. Without this energy, the cell will deteriorate, which may eventually lead to degenerative or chronic disease, though these may not become diagnosable or symptomatic for up to 25 years later. Weak electric fields also slow or halt injury recovery and healthy cell replacement.

health for everyone. While conventional western (allopathic) medicine primarily treats disease symptoms, most CAM methods aim at boosting the body's ability to heal itself through the immediate and long-term improvement of the immune system. Many chronic diseases, including some cancers, are now also thought to be caused by infectious agents. Therefore, a robust immune system is the first line of defense against these agents.

"I Sleep Here!"

HOW THE NYVATEX HEALTH-MAT™ WORKS

The Nyvatex Health-Mat generates the natural earth-equivalent electric field by triboelectrification—a process of electric charge separation that involves the rubbing together (friction) of dissimilar material surfaces. The triboelectric series is a classification method in electric theory for creating an electric field by friction rubbing. This patented design creates a natural electric field equivalent to the earth's electric field. The detailed physical mechanism in triboelectrification is a long unsolved problem, even with modern-day physics. ("Triboelectrification" is from the Greek word "tribo" [rubbing] and the English "electric.") The Nyvatex Health-Mat provides a solution and is the first practical patented tool employing this phenomenon. This patented discovery was to make it equivalent to and boost the earth's natural electric field, in which the human body thrives. No magnets, chemicals, drugs, batteries, or electric wires are used in the Nyvatex Health-Mat.

On May 9, 2006, some impressive mice with strong immune systems were reported on in the prestigious Proceedings of the National Academy of Sciences by researchers at Wake Forest University. The mice were resistant to injections of cancer cells that killed all ordinary mice. Even better, the researchers say, when white blood cells from these stronger mice were injected into non-resistant mice with cancerous tumors, the tumors vanished. The white blood cells from these cancer-immune mice were of types that confer innate immunity. They were naive as opposed to adaptive white blood cells, meaning they did not have to be exposed to the cancer cells in the first place to do their cancer-fighting job. Our Nyvatex Health-Mat has been shown in a national university biotech lab to increase naive T-cell proliferation by 55%.

While sleeping on our health mat, you will be bathing your body in the exact equivalent of the earth's natural electric field throughout the night. By taking part in the natural healing CAM therapies of your choice, and by eating high-energy live foods and supplements, you will be improving your body's immune function and its DNA-repairing ability by boosting its electric-energy field and conductivity.

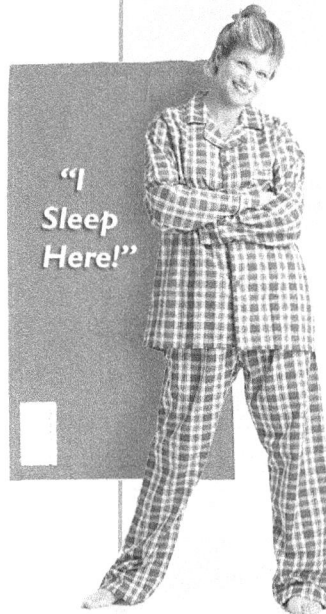

JOHN C. LEDBETTER is CEO of the Nyvatex Oil Corporation in Billings, Montana. He graduated from West Point in 1957, and served in the Army's Air Defense Missile Command. After eight high-tech years on Wall Street, he traveled extensively to test his proprietary, oil-finding inventions based on earth's radiation patterns. He began to see the health implications of his experiments with chaos mechanics (deep-pattern non-linear dynamics) for oil and gas exploration.

He applied his understanding to answer the confounding question, "Why are some people usually healthy no matter how they abuse their health, while others are sickly no matter how virtuously they take care of their health?" He noticed defined population areas with generally good health and others with poor health. He figured the difference had to do with where and how they lived.

His work with earth radiation patterns to locate subsurface oil provided the central clue, which led to the development of his health mat. His theories connect the Eastern *chi* therapies with Western electric-field science, considering these two energies to be one and the same—a healing force now easily accessible through the Nyvatex Health-Mat.

AUTHOR'S NOTE: Since this was published, John Ledbetter has since closed his company, so unfortunately, the health mat is not available. His research is reprinted here as a testament to his science and his integrity.

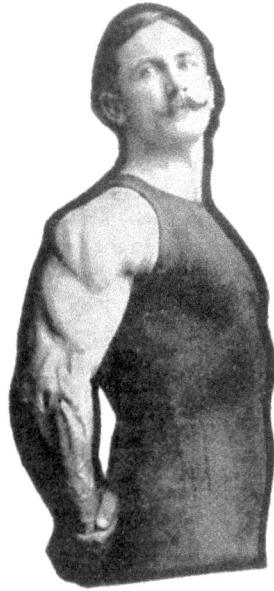

32nd Edition (320,000)

Price, 10 Cents

Deep

Breathing

By

Paul von Boeckmann, R. S.
103 Park Avenue
New York

Copyright, 1911, by P. von Boeckmann.

EDITOR'S NOTE: The following excerpts from Paul von Boeckmann were written almost 100 years ago. This material and the foregoing recommendation by Dr. D.O. Harrell are reprinted here with original illustrations as a tribute to this early exponent of good breathing and to honor the relevance of his writings today. There are a few inaccuracies; for instance, the concept that carbon dioxide is a poison, and some hyperbole, but his concepts were correct for the most part, especially considering his day and age. In *Deep Breathing*, he defends himself against those who called him a "breathing quack." Also included are excerpts from *Nerve Force*, which he wrote seven years later.

In our Integral Breathwork Seminars, we use von Boeckmann's three exercises for chest and lung expansion with good results (see next pages). Many of his conclusions coincide with current physiological understanding; yet much of what he taught, especially his emphasis on diaphragmatic breathing, is still not generally known today. (Note on the *Deep Breathing* cover, above, the number of editions printed and the number of copies sold by 1911!)

Von Boeckmann started off as a physical culturist. After learning from a breath-volume test that his lung capacity was far below normal, he spent the rest of his life studying about and developing his breathing, and teaching about good breathing for better health. ◼

Fatigue— Its Cause and Antidote

D.O. Harrell, MD

INTRODUCTION TO THE WORK OF PAUL VON BOECKMANN, PUBLISHED IN THE LITERARY DIGEST JANUARY 18, 1913

FATIGUE means poison.

Every muscular and nervous impulse causes the burning of vital fuel, and the ashes resulting are expelled along with carbon dioxide. Fatigue is simply an indication of an excess of this waste material in the system.

Another strange fact is that the ashes dumped into the blood by the waste of a muscle cell are exactly the same character as the ashes that are produced by a nerve cell or a brain cell. Hence, anything that tires the brain also tires the muscles, and vice versa.

This phenomenon has been clearly proven by Professor Fred Schiller Lee of Columbia College, expert on fatigue; and also by Dr. Maggiora of Turin, Italy. It is evident how useless it is to attempt to revive a tired brain through physical exercise as is so often recommended. According to Maggiora, rest and breathing are the only sensible antidotes for fatigue.

The foregoing facts should be kept vividly in the minds of everyone. Fatigue is a danger signal. It is an indication that your lungs have failed to throw off carbon dioxide as fast as it has accumulated. It is Nature's command to rest and breathe. There is no other cure for fatigue. It is through the lungs alone that this accumulated poison can be cast off. Endurance, whether mental, nervous, or muscular, is governed directly by the degree of your respiratory power.

Brain workers who lack power of mental concentration, who have a poor memory, or who become rapidly fatigued should ask themselves whether their system is not saturated with poison. Those who become fatigued rapidly through physical exertion may be sure that they too are suffering from the same poison.

This fatigue and lack of mental power is not due, as many wish to believe, to lack of proper or sufficient food. Most of us eat enough food to nourish a body and brain twice as large as that which we have. But not one person in a hundred breathes sufficiently to properly burn the food he eats or to throw off the ashes that result.

It is a lamentable fact that few persons know how to breathe or know the first laws of respiration. As long as they are not actually consumptives, they blindly assure themselves that they have large and active lungs.

There has come to my notice recently a book entitled *Deep Breathing*, by Paul von Boeckmann, RS. This treatise is by far the most sensible and valuable work I have ever read on the vital subject of breathing. The author is evidently a man of great experience and practical ideas.

I believe this booklet gives you the real key to constitutional strength. It shows us plainly how to develop a high degree of respiratory power so that we may cast off fatigue poison and other health destroying matter. It explains for the first time the danger of developing the external body at the expense of the internal body. The theories must be based on vast experience.

Personally, I know that his teachings are profoundly scientific and thoroughly practical, for I have had occasion to see them tested in a number of my patients.

The booklet to which I refer can be obtained from the author directly upon payment of ten cents in coin or stamps. The simple exercises he describes therein are worth many times the small price asked for the booklet.

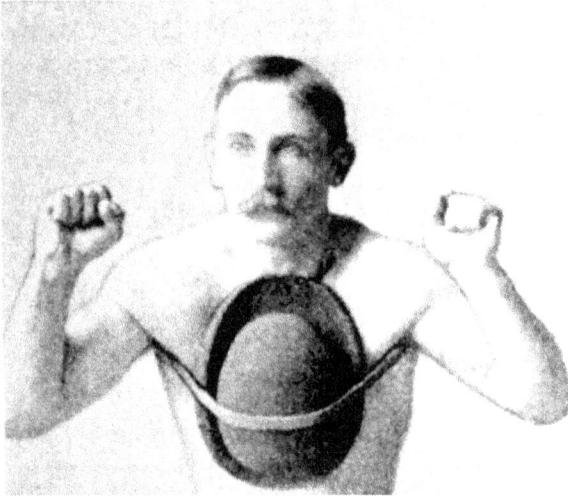

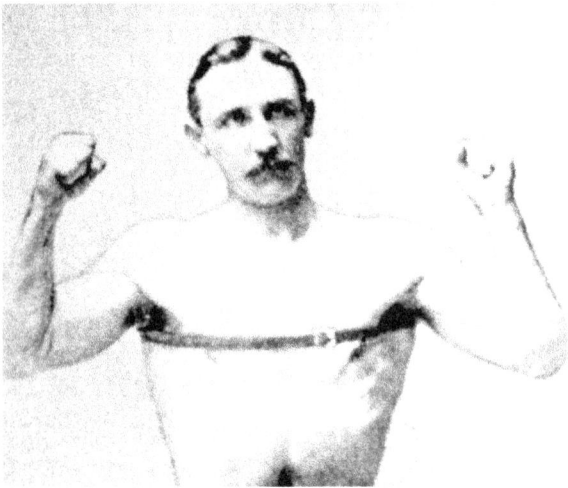

Paul von Boeckmann (1871–1944), health instructor in New York City, was well known to followers of physical culture in the early 1900s. Though in his youth he had been a strongman and a professional cyclist, he became much better known later as an instructor, particularly as an expert on lung development and deep breathing.

As the result of special attention to breathing exercises and to daily practice on a spirometer, von Boeckmann attained extraordinary lung power and a chest expansion of 11.5 inches. During this period, his lung or "vital" capacity increased from 180 cubic inches—a poor figure even to start with—to an eventual measurement of 436 inches, which at the time was surpassed only by the world record of 460 cubic inches. This was set in 1893.

Von Boeckmann demonstrated his chest expansion (as shown) by putting a belt around his chest, letting the air out of his lungs, then putting a derby hat inside the belt. Next, removing the hat and fully expanding his chest, he would fill out the space just occupied by the hat.

One of von Boeckmann's claims to fame was his tremendous grip strength. A lost relic of the Iron Game is von Boeckmann's Iron Indian Club, said to have tipped the scales at 80 pounds and standing approximately 20 inches high. Von Boeckmann grasped this club at the small end with his hands close together (in baseball bat style) and could readily lever it up and over his shoulder. He challenged many a strongman to lift the club. Eugene Sandow tried but failed to make the lift. Charles Atlas, with great effort, managed to lift it slightly once. Von Boeckmann also was able to chin himself for three repetitions using only the middle finger of his right hand. ▓

—*The Super Athletes* (1970) by David P. Willoughby

EDITOR'S NOTE: Von Boeckmann wrote several booklets and coached 60,000 high-school students on breathing in his lifetime. He uses the title—*Nerve Force*—in the booklet excerpted here (coming up in four pages). Back 100 years ago, Western medicine and physiology had no concept of the life-force energy running through the meridians (i.e., *prana, chi,* etc.). Yet he observed it and used Nerve Force to describe it: "We know this Nerve Force. It is the dominant power of our existence. It governs our whole life. It is Life. If we understood what Nerve Force is, we would know the secret of life." Here's his partial list of behaviors that *deplete* nerve force: Arguing, suspicion, grief, self-torture, worry, gossip, jealousy, impatience, lack of sleep, abuse of sex, and "nerve shocks" (i.e., trauma, PTSD). ▓

EXCERPTS FROM
Deep Breathing

Paul von Boeckmann, RS
circa 1911

Breathing is the Vital Force of Life. Air is the most important factor in the process of regenerating the vital forces. You cannot live five minutes without air. Almost instant death would result from oxygen starvation and the poisoning of every cell in the body.

The breathing organ is the great scavenger system. Enough deadly poison is thrown off by the lungs daily to kill a dozen elephants.

When one breathes fully and correctly, the black venous blood, foul with the ashes of burned brain cells and the debris of worn-out tissues, is transformed by the lungs at every breath into pure red blood.

We are a race of weak-lunged beings. The majority of persons breathe merely enough to keep alive. The present-day mile-a-minute life requires extraordinarily strong lungs and breathing power.

Develop your lungs commensurate with the demands that are placed upon them, which are very great. Do not be a victim of colds, short-windedness, thin blood, and a thousand and one ailments that are due to shallow and improper breathing.

All animals and man, except when under severe strain, breathe diaphragmatically. When it becomes necessary to breathe extraordinary volumes of air, chest respiration is employed. When large quantities of oxygen are needed, and when an excess of muscular and nervous refuse is being dumped into the blood, we must breathe by the chest method.

Diaphragmatic breathing causes a circulation of air through a larger area of lung tissue than does chest breathing. This permits the blood to absorb more oxygen and cast off more carbon dioxide.

Chest breathing, by virtue of the fact that it demands the bending and raising of the ribs, requires considerable expenditure of muscular and nervous energy, while this expenditure is very low with diaphragmatic breathing. Only the soft and yielding sections of the trunk need be expanded.

Diaphragmatic breathing is the natural method employed habitually by all healthy human beings and animals. The diaphragm is the muscle that pumps the lungs. When this muscle becomes weak and inactive, oxygen starvation results, the blood becomes less purified, and the internal organs do not receive the massaging motion they require to maintain their functions.

With each breath, blood is made to circulate through the organs of digestion, absorption, and elimination. The stomach and liver lie just beneath and adjacent to that powerful breathing muscle, the diaphragm, hence receiving direct massaging and kneading. I believe this diaphragmatic massage is one of the most important physiological acts of the human organism.

Abundant pure air is the most powerful tonic known in nature. Artificial tonics (drugs) are poisons—stimulants that whip up jaded nerves

The Lungs and Chest

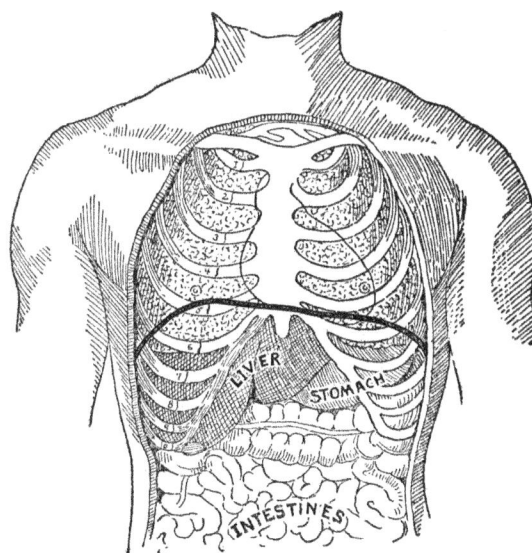

Fig. 3
CHART SHOWING THE FORMATION OF THE TRUNK, AND RELATIVE POSITION OF THE VITAL ORGANS. THE HORIZONTAL BLACK LINE REPRESENTS THE DIAPHRAGM.

and tired muscles just as a cruel driver whips up a weak and sick horse into a trot. Combine deep breathing with rational exercise and you will experience real vigor, real snap and vivacity. Beware of "drug tonics."

Next to deep breathing, the most important hygienic measure is light physical exercise. Exercise promotes the circulation of the blood, gives tone and elasticity to the muscles, and preserves the coordination between the brain and the muscles. Rest, recreation, sleep, and cleanliness also play important roles in health. Forceful breathing brings into play many of the most powerful groups of muscles of the body—muscles which play the main role in the preservation of good health. Two hours devoted to deep breathing and exercise a week is sufficient to prolong one's life at least ten years. Thus, four days of bodily care means a year added to one's life. A paltry 9,000% interest on your investment!

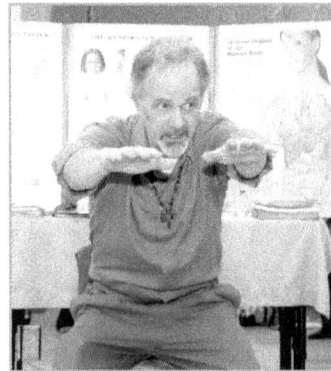

Denis attempting to demonstrate Exercise B, at a seminar in 20017, in Bozeman, MT.

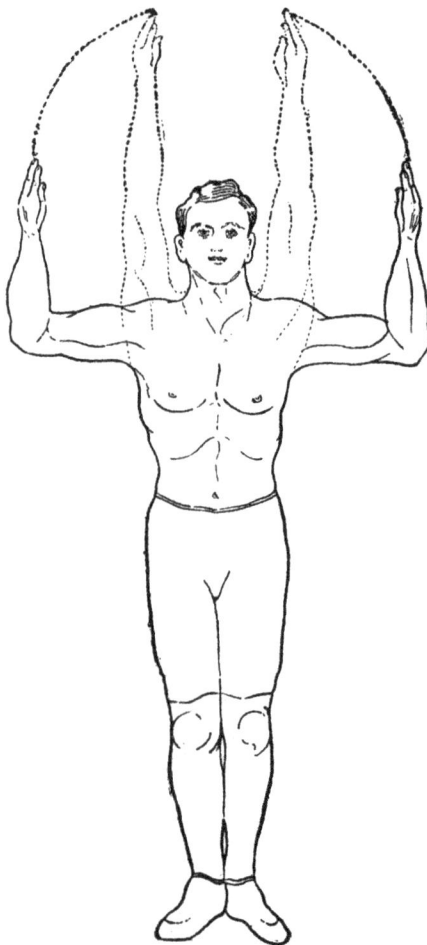

Chart A

Breathing Exercise A

Starting Position: Assume the position shown in solid line.

First Movement: Raise the body to an erect position and extend the arms over the head as indicated by the dotted line. A chest inhalation should be taken during the movement. Duration of inhalation and movement should be five seconds.

Second Movement: Exhale and drop arms to the sides.

This exercise should be repeated from 5 to 10 times, at intervals of about 15 seconds, alternating the position of the feet. That is, first perform the exercise with the left foot forward, and then with the right foot forward.

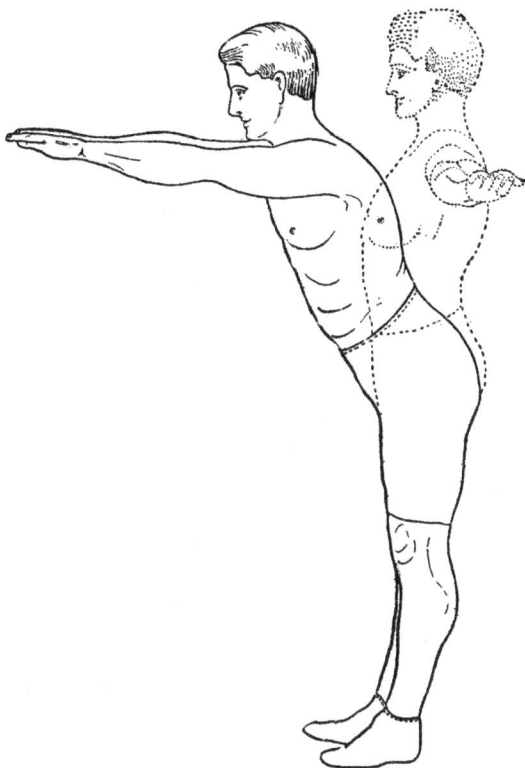

Chart B

Breathing Exercise B

Starting Position: Assume the position as indicated by solid lines, arms extended forward and palms turned downward, as shown.

First Movement: Raise the body to the erect position and fling the arms backward as indicated by the dotted lines. The turning of palms takes place near the end of the movement.
A deep chest inhalation is taken during the exercise. The duration of the movement and inhalation should be about three seconds.

Second Movement: Exhale and drop arms to the sides.

This exercise should be repeated from 8 to 12 times at intervals of 10 seconds.

Breathing Exercise C

Starting Position: Assume the position as shown in solid line.

First Movement: Take a deep chest inhalation and while doing so stretch the arms slowly above the head until they reach the position shown by dotted lines. Be sure to stretch the arms to the greatest height. The duration of inhalation and movement should take about three seconds.

Second Movement: Exhale and return arms to starting position shown in solid line.

This exercise should be repeated from 10 to 20 times at intervals of five seconds.

It is highly important that the movement of the arms be in perfect rhythm with the inhalation and exhalation. Observing this instruction will develop the coordination between the brain and the breathing muscles. Therefore, do not complete the inhalation before the hands have been raised to the highest point. The respiratory movement and arm movement should begin together and end together. Observe this rule in Exercises B and C.

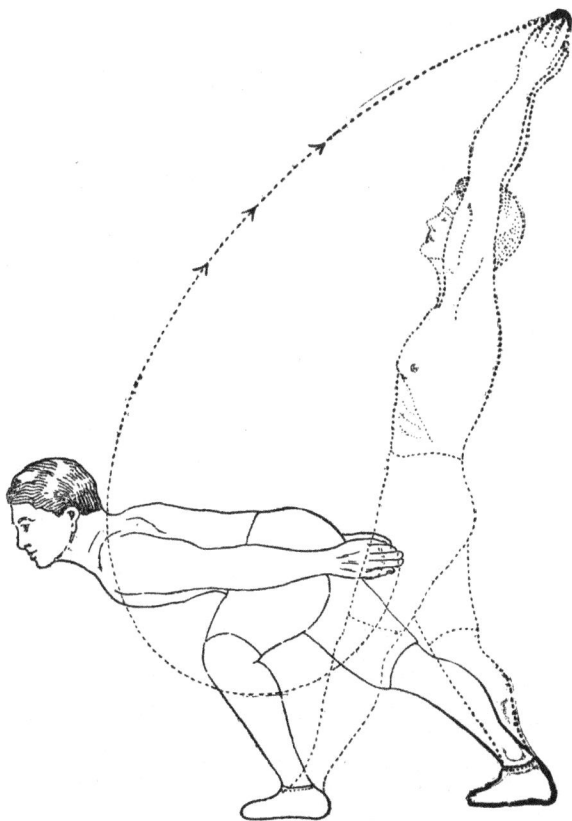

Chart C

EXCERPTS FROM

Nerve Force

Paul von Boeckmann, RS
circa 1918

BREATHING

The power of the vital organs depends directly upon the nerve stimulus they receive from the nervous system. Nerve exhaustion impairs the action of the stomach, bowels, and other abdominal organs, causing endless distress and ailments. The heart and lungs are especially affected through nerve exhaustion and nerve tension. We have all observed that the slightest excitement will cause the heart to beat rapidly and breathing to increase. Fear and worry depress the action of the heart and lungs. This depression is very injurious.

The heart and lungs may be considered a single organ, the Master Organ of the Body, upon which life depends more directly than upon the other organs. When the heart stops beating, death will result in a few minutes. In other words, the blood is the Stream of Life, which must be kept flowing freely through the body, and it must be kept pure. It is the duty of the heart and lungs to do this. With each breath, life-giving oxygen is carried to the blood, and poisons are carried off along with carbon dioxide. It is highly essential, therefore, that first of all, we breathe deeply. Next in importance is that we breathe correctly. I shall describe here the two principal methods of breathing, namely, chest breathing and diaphragmatic breathing.

CHEST BREATHING

Chest breathing means that form of breathing which results from the movement of the rib section of the trunk, especially the upper section of the chest. That is, during inhalation the chest expands; and during exhalation it contracts. This form of breathing, especially when performed to the limit of exhalation and inhalation, is an excellent form of internal exercise and develops the size of the chest, which is beneficial in many ways.

DIAPHRAGMATIC BREATHING

Diaphragmatic breathing, sometimes called abdominal breathing, is entirely different in action from chest breathing. During inhalation the abdomen expands, and during exhalation the abdomen contracts. It must be understood that air does not enter the abdominal region in this form of breathing. This is impossible. By referring to the accompanying diagram, the mechanical action will be readily understood. The curved line (A) represents the diaphragm, the broad muscle that separates the heart and lungs from the abdominal organs. When this muscle descends, it causes suction within the chest cavity, causing an inflow of air into the lungs (inhalation). When the diaphragm rises, air is forced out of the lungs (exhalation).

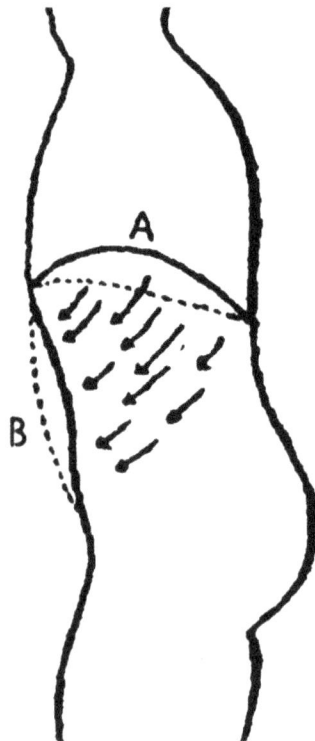

The alternate rise and fall of this muscle causes a corresponding movement of the abdominal organs, thus causing the abdomen to expand and contract as described. This causes an alternate high and low pressure within the abdominal cavity.

Diaphragmatic breathing is the proper method in tranquil breathing, whereas chest breathing is employed only during strenuous exertion. As an exercise, diaphragmatic breathing may be termed normal breathing, while chest breathing is a form of forced breathing, just as a forced draft may be applied to a boiler in case great steam pressure is needed.

It may seem strange that breathing, an act we perform from the beginning of life to the very end, could be done otherwise than correctly, but we need only observe our fellow men to see evidence that few people breathe diaphragmatically at all times. Instead, they usually breathe by the chest method. As babes and children we all breathe correctly, but later, because of the clothing we wear and the cramped positions we assume in sitting, the action of the diaphragm is restricted, thus compelling the more powerful chest muscles to come to the rescue. This gradually promotes the habit of chest breathing. Years of practice of this habit permit it to become so deep-seated that it requires much patient effort to correct it.

ADVANTAGES OF DIAPHRAGMATIC BREATHING

Diaphragmatic breathing has certain great advantages over chest breathing. In the first place, it compels air to enter mainly into the lower and larger sections of the lungs, thus promoting greater blood oxygenation. Another important advantage is that the alternate high and low pressure in the abdominal cavity stimulates the circulation of blood in that region, which is so very essential in the proper action of the vital organs.

Diaphragmatic breathing stimulates an action known as peristalsis, a worm-like motion of the intestines and bowels, which promotes digestion and the elimination of waste matter. I know of thousands of cases where a change from chest to diaphragmatic breathing corrected long-standing cases of constipation, indigestion, liver trouble, etc.

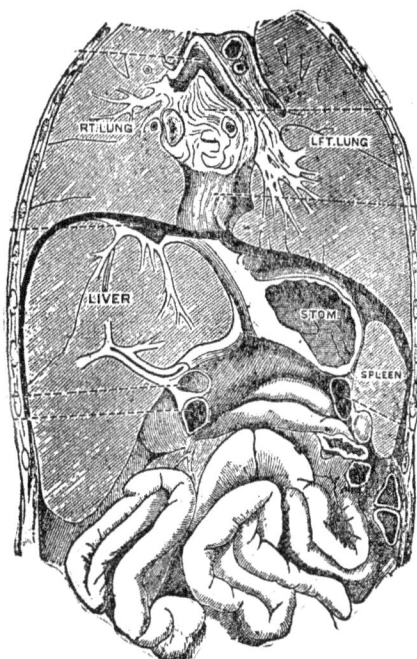

Fig. 2
FRONT VIEW (SECTIONAL)
THE HORIZONTAL BLACK LINE REPRESENTS
THE DIAPHRAGM

ITS EFFECT ON THE NERVES

Diaphragmatic breathing has a remarkable effect upon the pneumo-gastric nerve and especially upon the solar plexus. It breaks up the paralyzing nerve tension so often observed in people with supersensitive and deranged nerves.

The close relation existing among the pneumo-gastric nerve, breathing, and the vital organs is demonstrated when a baby is born. In an unborn babe the vital organs are practically at a standstill. If food were in the stomach it would not be digested, but with the first breath, the *breath of life*, the entire vital machinery is set in motion. This breath means the awakening of the pneumo-gastric nerve and especially the solar plexus.

HOW TO BEGIN

A good plan is to begin practicing diaphragmatic breathing while lying down, for it is most easily performed when in this position. After faithful practice for a few weeks, it may be practiced while sitting or standing, until finally full control will be attained over the diaphragm, and in time it will become an unconscious habit.

Conscious diaphragmatic breathing is of great value in restoring the heart action to normal. Heart fluttering, skipping of beats, and other abnormal manifestations in heart action are very common in people with deranged nerves. I know of many cases where diaphragmatic breathing greatly helped most serious forms of so-called heart trouble. The inculcation of the habit of diaphragmatic breathing should therefore be one of the first aims in everyone, be he a victim of nerve conditions or not. ▪

The Continuum

Parting Thoughts • *Denis Ouellette*

Chalchas, priest of Apollo, reading the omens from the liver of a sacrificed sheep, based on an episode in Homer's *Iliad*. This mythical Greek *haruspex* (soothsayer) is represented here in the Etruscan (pre-Roman) iconographic version with wings, a characteristic that underlines his function as intercessor between earthly and transcendental reality. The foot placed on a rock is a fundamental action in the divining process. In doing this he establishes contact with the earth as the site of the natural sphere and the underworld. The image below was drawn on an etching plate in 1974, from a photo of the original Etruscan engraved bronze mirror from 400 BC. Vatican Gregorian Etruscan Museum. The inscription reads *Xalxas*.

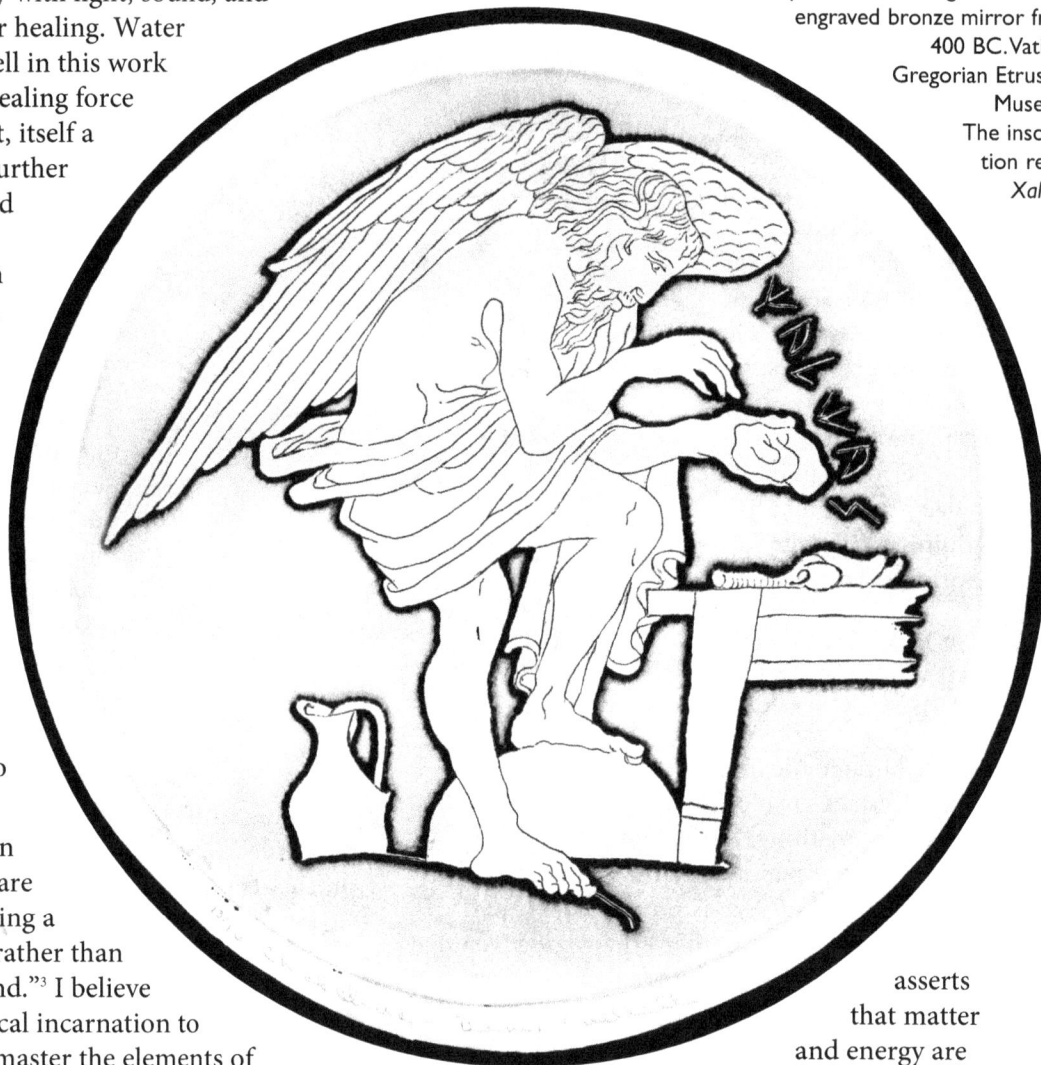

We have explored using the breath in harmony with light, sound, and water for healing. Water complements air well in this work and carries a vital healing force of its own.[1] Sunlight, itself a potent healer, can further charge the water and heal your body.[2] Spiritual energy can be invoked through chanting sacred syllables. Worded invocations spoken with visualization and intent employ subtler qualities of light and etheric color rays that interact with the chakras and bring their specific gifts and qualities to the healing work.

Author Dannion Brinkley says, "We are spiritual beings having a human experience rather than the other way around."[3] I believe we come into physical incarnation to understand and to master the elements of earth, air, fire, and water, and the pranic life-forces moving within each of them. When we go beyond this life, we take this learning with us for the greater creative endeavors that await us. It's as though these elements in their marvelous inter-play here on earth were created with this hidden yet pivotal purpose in mind—to teach us, to heal us, and to assist us in transcending ourselves.

We live within a vibrational continuum from matter to energy. Einstein's relativity theory asserts that matter and energy are interchangeable. Atomic theory describes matter while quantum theory describes energy in its many forms: heat, light, sound, electricity, etc. Quantum physics takes us deep into matter to show us that, at the most fundamental level, all matter is energy. Everything that surrounds us lies somewhere along an energetic continuum, vibrating at different frequencies. The slower the wave-lengths, the denser the matter.

Scientists say that the primal particles produced by the Big Bang were not atoms, nor were they protons, neutrons, or electrons, but the basic constituents of all of these, which they call quarks. No quarks have ever been seen in the laboratory because, according to theory, they cannot exist as free particles. There's no proof that quarks exist, but because they explain best how atoms behave, most physicists believe in them. (Scientists taking a leap of faith!)

> *In the universe there is an immeasurable, indescribable force which shamans call intent, and absolutely everything that exists in the entire cosmos is attached to intent by a connecting link.*
>
> —Carlos Castaneda

An essential underpinning of quantum physics is that there is no separation between subject and object, the observer and the observed. Particles of energy seen through an electron microscope behave in a manner that is expected of them by the observer. Thus no separation is apparent between the matter particle and the thought or intent of the observer.

As we move higher still in vibration along the continuum, beyond energy and thought, we come to the contemplation of what Wallace Wattles, in 1910, called "the Formless Living Substance."[4] It's what Wayne Dyer calls the Source and the "field of intention" that surrounds us. This pure energy is supercharged by its Creator to carry an intent toward Light, Life and Love. This accounts for the powerful, undeniable force within us, and within all of nature, to grow and to expand, to seek wholeness and to keep transforming until the ultimate intended design—the blueprint—within the DNA, within our souls, within the acorn is reached. The ancient maxim of Hermes Trismegistus comes to mind, *As Above* (in the divine intent), *So Below* (in manifestation).

By its nature, energy wants to follow our creative thoughts and feelings. When a destructive direction is taken, the impersonal result is Life dying, Light dimming, and Love disappearing. Our understanding of this law is innate, because the thrust of this energy is what drives us. So it's not difficult to catch the wave and ride it for our healing. More difficult is *kicking against the pricks*[5]—going against the flow. When we set our intent persistently toward Light, Life and Love, everything in creation, from quarks to elemental forces to our emotions, our thoughts, and our physical health, *conspires* to help us. (Doesn't that word also mean "to breathe with?")

The elements have their correspondences inside of us. Thus earth is said to be our physical body, air our mental body, water our emotional body, and fire our memory body. Since we live along all of this continuum at once, let's approach our healing holistically rather than separating, compartmentalizing, and specializing, as we in the West are predisposed to do. The elements of our nature all intermingle and deeply affect each other. There is no separating them. When one is healed, the others are also; when one is damaged, the others are too.

> *That which is Below corresponds to that which is Above, and that which is Above corresponds to that which is Below, to accomplish the miracles of the One Thing. And just as all things have come from this One Thing, through the meditation of One Mind, so do all created things originate from this One Thing, through Transformation.*
>
> —*The Emerald Tablet* of Hermes Trismegistus

Natural healing is always done slowly and gently and is never forced. The dramatic stories you've read from people doing this work came about in their own time, when the people were ready. Most people come to healing work just wanting some relief from pain or stress—they want to feel better. Breathwork is a great starting point because the life-force within oxygen is powerfully apparent and vitally essential.

Breathwork helps you shed the burdens of your past, including physical toxins and mental and emotional patterning. It will unlock and resolve memories that you no longer need to carry around. It will help you enjoy life more and fulfill your own goals and purposes better. Breathwork can be taught simply from the point of view of improving health, relieving stress, and oxygenating and detoxing your body. If people emerge from a breathwork session feeling peaceful, energized, and ready to face their world, we have done our job well.

Eventually, once the heavier burdens are gone, breathwork will bring people face-to-face with their spiritual nature, whatever that means for them, whenever they're ready. The more prana you let in, the more of spirit you let in. One day, you look around (and you look within) and spirit is all you see. You are still aware of all the disparate energies along the continuum, even the human struggles and negativities, but they are in perspective and you look upon them with compassion.

Starting your journey with breathwork is a good opening move in the direction toward wholeness. The Integral Breathwork format we have introduced in this book is a sound, wise, and grounded approach. It can work well for you. Others may gravitate to accessing their energy through yoga, fasting, hydrotherapy, the oriental *chi* disciplines or martial arts, nature-based or traditional religions, even sun gazing.

The world's cultures are rich with arts and sciences that can also lead to marvelous awak-

> Intention is a power that's present everywhere as a field of energy; it isn't limited to physical development. It's the source of nonphysical development, too. This field of intention is here, now, and available to you. When you activate it, you'll begin to feel purpose in your life, and you'll be guided by your infinite self.... As *you* make your metaphorical bow to this power, recognize that you're bowing to yourself. The all-pervading energy of intention pulses through you toward your potential for a purposeful life.
>
> —Dr. Wayne W. Dyer,
> *The Power of Intention*

enings of self-discovery. Ask any creative genius. From athletics to academics, from business to family life, spirit dwells at all points along the continuum. Any endeavor with the underlying intent toward Light, Life and Love will yield its rewards. When this intent is set, it's not as if you even need to decide the course; you're following the electron stream. The Taoists would call this being "in the *tao*." This book came to you, and you got this far in reading it, because there's something here for you. Why not give this therapeutic approach a try.

Spirit is free. Air, fire, water, and earth are all freely given as the platform of our life, but they contain secret messages, hidden energy keys to unlocking your healing and transformation. Can you divine their inner power and meaning like our friend Chalchas? The hidden plan is to give you far more than you ever knew was possible. *It is your Father's good pleasure to give you the kingdom!*[6] So embrace the vast and varied continuum of your true nature. All of it is good—all is God.

1. Study Father Sebastian Kneipp's pioneering work with naturopathy, holistic health, and hydrotherapy at www.Kneipp.com.

2. For more on using solar energy for self-healing, see the work of both Hira Ratan Manek (1937–present) at www.SolarHealing.com; and the inspiring life of Omraam Mikhaël Aïvanhov (1900–1986) at www.FrankPerry.co.uk/aivanhov.htm or www.Prosveta.com.

3. Dannion Brinkley, author of *Saved by the Light* and other books. Visit www.Dannion.com.

4. Wallace D. Wattles, *The Science of Getting Rich*

5. Reference to Acts 9:5.

6. Reference to Luke 12:32.

CHAPTER	**APPENDIX**

30. OPTIMAL BREATHING

Optimal Breathing Self-Test, Parts 1 & 2 — 150

Supporting a More Optimal Breathing Pattern:

   The Pear, the Cone & the Wave • *Squeeze & Breathe Exercise* — 154

31. INTEGRAL BREATHWORK

Seminar Flyers, Agenda, Registration Packet & Evaluation Form — 156

Our Nervous Systems — 162

What to Do • *What to Expect* — 166

Goal Setting — 168

Seven Chakras & Associations • Illustration — 170

	RESOURCES

32. RESOURCES

Recommended Reading & Suggested Music — 172

Healing Art of Conscious Breathing CD User's Guide—John Meneghini — 174

E3Live*: Earth's First Food*—Michael Saiber — 176

Zap-A-Kramp: Nature's Solution to Cramping & Tetany—Carlton Newman — 180

NaturalLifeNews.com — 181

Natural Life News & Directory — 182

OPTIMAL BREATHING® SELF-TEST ~ PART 1

PHYSICAL ASSESSMENTS & MEASUREMENTS

Use the form at right to log your progress. Explanations and statistics are in bold below.

A. Upper Chest Expansion Measurement

Have a friend assist you. Take a cloth tape measure and wrap it around your upper chest as high up into your armpits as you can. Exhale fully and measure the girth. Then inhale fully and measure the girth. Note the difference between the two measurements.

- *This measures rib flexibility. The rib, chest, and shoulder muscles play almost as important a part in lung squeezing as does the diaphragm.*

- *Some insurance companies use this measurement to gauge longevity and insurability.*

- *Between 1" and 2" is average. From 3" to 4" is good.*

- *If you are 5'2", one inch is not great, but it is OK. For someone of this height, 3.5" is excellent.*

- *If you are 6'2", less than 2" is not great. For someone of this height, 4.25" is excellent.*

B. Buddy Observations: Unbalanced Deep Breathing (UDB)

Ask someone to observe you. While standing, take a very deep breath—as deep as you can. When you breathe in very deeply:

1. Do you raise your rib cage?
2. Do you raise your shoulders?
3. Do your neck muscles bulge out?

- *The diaphragm and rib cage should do the breathing.*

- *Neither your shoulders nor rib cage should move upward. (The ribs should expand outward, not upward.)*

- *Your neck muscles should not bulge out at all.*

C. Belly or Chest Breather?

Place one hand on your chest, and one on your belly. Breathe in. Which expands first? Assign percentages (60 chest/40 belly).

- *Chest expanding first indicates UDB or reverse breathing. This is one of the worst ways to breathe because it over-stimulates the nervous system, inviting anxiety, hyperventilation, acidic blood, heart stress, and other maladies. Ideal is 70% belly.*

D. Complete Breaths per Minute

Sit comfortably. A complete breath is one inhale and one exhale, plus a pause at the end of the exhale. How many complete breaths did you have in one minute? If you are unsure of the count, repeat the number count test 2–3 times or until the last number count is identical or nearly the same as the one before it.

- *The more times per minute you breathe, the higher the stress and oxygen cost. Higher breathing rates carry over into sleep time and relate to excessive stress responses, anxiety, heart conditions, high blood pressure, strokes, and far less than optimal health. They help cause or worsen every health condition known to mankind.*

15 or more	=	Poor
11–14	=	Fair
8–10	=	Good
6–7	=	Very Good
5	=	Excellent

E. Breathing Pause

The length of time—in seconds or half seconds—at the end of an exhale before the next inhale. Follow your breathing and note in your mind, or have a friend keep time for you, the length of the pause at the end of a natural, effortless exhale. "One thousand one, two thousand two, three thousand three" is three seconds. "One thou-" would be a half second. So "one thousand one, two thousand two, three thou-" equals 2.5 seconds.

- *The pause is the resting phase between the out-breath and the in-breath. No pause = no rest for the nervous system. With too short a pause, your body never really rests.*

- *Like a car engine, you either are running at high RPMs all the time and on too few cylinders, or you are idling low and running with plenty of power to spare.*

- *According to research, a pause of less than 2.5 seconds definitely requires improvement and lengthening of the pause.*

- *With a pause that is less than one second, your nervous system is always in a state of emergency. And you've got some serious work to do.*

F. Breathing Pause Extension

Let a natural exhale occur. At the bottom or end of a natural exhale, resist breathing in as long as you can. Time it in seconds.

- *Recent research in Russia indicates a healthy minimum is 45 seconds. Higher is better—even up to 90 seconds.*

- *Below 45 seconds strongly indicates some kind of UDB or poor physical conditioning.*

- *Anything less than 30 seconds may accompany shortness of breath or asthma.*

G. Breathing Volume & Oxygen Uptake Efficiency

Sit with back straight. Take as large an in-breath as possible and then, as quietly and quickly as you can, count and still be heard—like a fast-talking auctioneer whispering—count up to as high a number as you can reach on this one full exhale. Note the number and try it again. Try it a third time if you think the number will be much different. *Do not* inhale during counting, skip any numbers, hold your breath, or breathe in and count at the same time. *Do* start again at 1 if you reach 100. Make sure you include the beginnings of each number such as the thirty in thirty-three. Repeat the tests in the same position you were in for the previous tests. OK, try it now. How high a number did you reach in that one long exhaled breath? Perform this again and write down the average of the two.

- *Below 100. Research strongly indicates that if the count is below 100, you may have a serious health challenge or unbalanced deep breathing (UDB) that can invite one.*

- *100–200 indicates something is probably off, or there is a tendency for some manner of health issue to occur over time.*

- *200–250 is quite good; the person rarely if ever gets sick.*

- *Science has proven that your primary markers for longevity are breathing volume (Total Lung Capacity, TLC) and efficiency (flow rate as in Forced Exhalation Volume).*

BREATHING ASSESSMENTS

Name: _____

	Date:	Date:	Date:	Date:
A. Upper Chest Expansion Measurement				
Inches at complete INHALE:	_____	_____	_____	_____
Inches at complete EXHALE:	_____	_____	_____	_____
Difference between the two:	_____	_____	_____	_____
B. Buddy Observations:				
1. Do you raise your rib cage?	_____	_____	_____	_____
2. Do you raise your shoulders?	_____	_____	_____	_____
3. Do neck muscles bulge out?	_____	_____	_____	_____
C. Belly or Chest Breather? Place one hand on chest, one hand on belly. Breathe in....				
Which expands first? (circle one) and by what %? (60/40, etc.)	____/____ chest / belly	____/____ chest / belly	____/____ chest / belly	____/____ chest / belly
D. Complete Breaths Per Minute				
How many per minute?	_____	_____	_____	_____
E. Breathing Pause				
How many seconds (incl. 1/2)?	_____	_____	_____	_____
F. Breathing Pause Extension				
Seconds held at end of breath?	_____	_____	_____	_____
G. Breathing Volume & Oxygen Uptake Efficiency				
Highest Count, 1st time:	_____	_____	_____	_____
Highest Count, 2nd time:	_____	_____	_____	_____
Average of the two:	_____	_____	_____	_____

OPTIMAL BREATHING® SELF-TEST ~ PART 2

Check off these indicators as they apply to you. As you work on improving your breathing, recheck this list and note the changes that have occurred.

PHYSICAL RESTRICTIONS

Sit on the edge of a chair with your feet flat on the floor and legs hip-width apart. Close your eyes, go within, and take the deepest breath in and out that you can. Now take another deep in-and-out breath. Then allow yourself to breathe normally, and open your eyes. Did you experience one or more of the following conditions?

1. ❑ Unsatisfying or short breath
2. ❑ Can't catch breath or deep breathing curtailed
3. ❑ Breathing feels stuck
4. ❑ Feel a hitch, bump, or lump right below your breastbone when you try to take a deep breath
5. ❑ Breathing feels like a series of events instead of smooth, internally coordinated, and continuous
6. ❑ Breathing is labored or restricted
7. ❑ Breathing is shallow
8. ❑ Wheezing
9. ❑ Breathlessness, air hunger, or suffocation
10. ❑ Sigh or yawn often
11. ❑ Tightness, soreness, or pressure in the chest or below the breast bone
12. ❑ Sore, deep pain that feels like a band across the chest
13. ❑ Pulsing or stabbing feeling around the ribs
14. ❑ Side stitches
15. ❑ Chest wall tenderness
16. ❑ Chest feels large and stiff
17. ❑ Ribs flair outward at bottom during inhale
18. ❑ Cramps in belly or below sternum
19. ❑ Tense overall feeling
20. ❑ Tightness around the mouth

MENTAL SIGNALS

1. ❑ Poor memory
2. ❑ Negative attitude
3. ❑ Too many thoughts that will not stop when you would like them to
4. ❑ Confusion or sense of losing normal contact with surroundings
5. ❑ Light-headedness or "spaced out"
6. ❑ Disorientation
7. ❑ Dizzy spells
8. ❑ Black-out

EMOTIONAL SIGNALS

1. ❑ Anxiety
2. ❑ Apprehension
3. ❑ Phobias
4. ❑ Excessive shyness
5. ❑ Panic attacks
6. ❑ Emotional mood swings
7. ❑ Depression (chronic or mild)
8. ❑ Grief (repressed, unresolved)
9. ❑ Obsessive/compulsive behaviors
10. ❑ Addictions
11. ❑ Hypervigilance (jumpy)
12. ❑ Type-A personality (driven)
13. ❑ Excessive anger (abusive)

BODY SIGNALS

1. ❑ Chest pain
2. ❑ Mouth breather.
3. ❑ Chronic cough
4. ❑ Snoring
5. ❑ Hyperventilation
6. ❑ Often catch yourself not breathing
7. ❑ Waken from sleep or resting sud-

denly not breathing (sleep apnea)

8. ❏ Get tired from reading out loud
9. ❏ Sunken chest
10. ❏ Reduced pain tolerance
11. ❏ Chronic pain
12. ❏ Irregular heartbeats
13. ❏ Scoliosis or abnormal curvature of the spine
14. ❏ Excessive or frequent stress
15. ❏ High blood pressure
16. ❏ Hormonal fluctuations
17. ❏ Lump in throat
18. ❏ Jaw tension
19. ❏ Constipation
20. ❏ Upset stomach or irritable bowel syndrome
21. ❏ Reflux
22. ❏ Headaches
23. ❏ Sallow complexion

ENERGY

1. ❏ Energy is low
2. ❏ Wake up tired
3. ❏ Just want more energy
4. ❏ Want increased sexual energy
5. ❏ Blood sugar is low

SITTING POSITIONS

1. ❏ Drowsy when driving a vehicle
2. ❏ Often fall asleep while sitting up when you would rather have watched the program, heard the speaker, seen the game, etc.?
3. ❏ Get really bad jet lag
4. ❏ Sit in a car, bus, train, plane, or office chair more than a few hours daily

OPTIMAL BREATHING SIGNALS

1. ❏ Open, free, easy breathing in chest, sides, back, belly
2. ❏ Nostrils open and free
3. ❏ Never sick
4. ❏ Wake up refreshed
5. ❏ Steady-to-great energy all day
6. ❏ Quick recovery from physical exertion or stress
7. ❏ Good mood, positive can-do attitude
8. ❏ Clear-headed
9. ❏ Strong and free self-expression
10. ❏ Strong self-esteem
11. ❏ Healthy relationships (5 or more)
12. ❏ Breathing changes when communicating with loved ones about specific issues
13. ❏ Breathing changes when around specific people, places, or things

POSTURE—DO YOU SLOUCH AT ALL?

In other words, would you consider your posture to be less than excellent?

_____

_____

DESIRED LONGEVITY

Science has proven that your breathing quantity and quality largely control how long you will live. Imagine living a vibrantly healthy life. To what age do you wish to live?

_____

_____

Take the free breathing test online at www.Breathing.com and your statistics will be added to Mike White's database.

Supporting a More Optimal Breathing Pattern

The Pear (70%) **+ the Cone** (30%) **= the Wave** (100%)

SQUEEZE & BREATHE EXERCISE

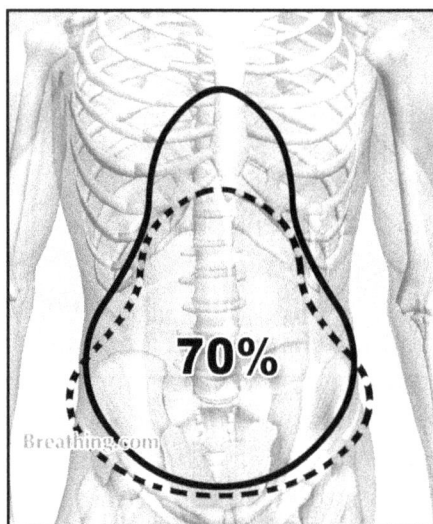

━━━━━━ **Exhale** (resting)

▬ ▬ ▬ ▬ **Inhale** (lungs full)

The Pear

Imagine a pear hanging from your collarbone. Your diaphragm lies on top of the lower portion of the pear. It rises and falls with each breath. At the end of an exhale, the diaphragm rests up inside your ribs in its natural dome shape. During an inhale, as your lungs fill, the top of the pear is pushed down and the diaphragm descends. This causes the lower, round part of the pear to expand in 360 degrees. The soft tissue of the abdomen will expand more than the sides (where your intercostal muscles are) and more than your lower back and kidney areas, but you should still feel expansion in your sides and back—although many do not, due to low-back tension. This primary *pear movement* should account for about 70% of the volume of your in-breath, since most of your lung tissue is in the lower half of your torso (and indeed the lungs hang down about 20% more toward the back like the tails on a tuxedo).

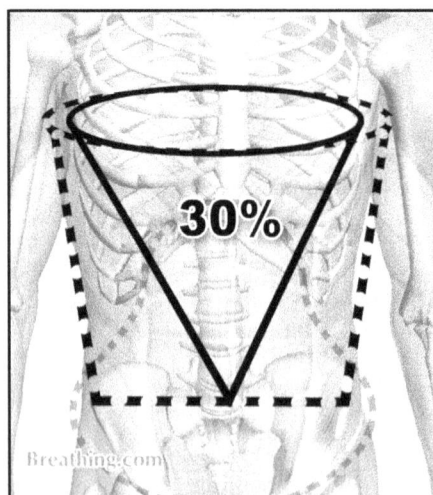

The Cone

Imagine a cone with the point anchored at your navel. The upper circle of the cone is approximately at the nipples. After the pear is filled, the breath will naturally rise up to open the ribs and expand the chest. This is the simultaneous secondary movement of the inhale, which accounts for about 30% of its volume. The pear and the cone enlarge as one, but the ribs do not expand until the lungs need more space for a deeper breath. The circle of the cone opens wider as the ribs spread sideways—but not upward.

Since the cone is anchored at the navel, it cannot lose its foundation. If the ribs were lifted during an inhale by shrugging the shoulders and bulging the neck muscles, the circle at the top of the cone might decrease in diameter, restricting your air volume intake.

(Imagine the tension you would accumulate from doing shoulder shrugs and tensing your neck muscles 15,000 to 35,000 times a day.) This might lead to reverse breathing, where the abdomen goes in during an inhale. The ideal is to keep your shoulders and neck at rest and allow your chest to widen sideways, with the ribs expanding from their two pivot points at the sternum and the spine. (There will be a gentle movement in the shoulders and the back of the neck as the inhale wave peaks.)

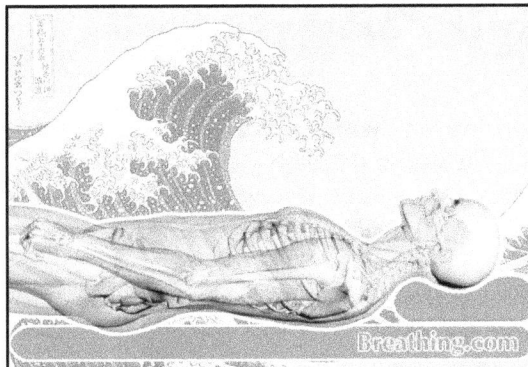

The Wave

The merging of the pear and cone as one continuous movement creates a marvelous wave that first fills the belly, then rises up the torso. You can harmonize the breath wave with the spinal wave. The gentle undulation of the spine will encourage the flow of spinal fluid, lubricating your spinal discs. Since the majority of your activity and attention should be in your lower torso, you will be stimulating the vagus nerve and the parasympathetic aspect of your autonomic nervous system. Like an ocean wave, when your inhale gets to its peak, it will spill its momentum on the shore. This is your free and relaxed exhale. You may feel inclined to pause before your next inhale, because you will be oxygenated and refreshed.

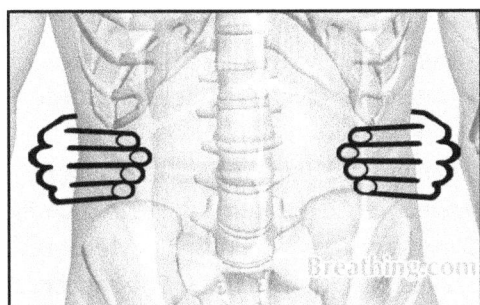

Squeeze & Breathe Exercise

To strengthen the diaphragm from within, perform the breath wave while placing a little extra pressure with your hands in the soft tissue between your hips and your ribs. Place your four fingers in the front and your thumbs in the back over your kidneys. Do this while standing with your feet shoulder-width apart, knees slightly bent, chin raised slightly above horizon level. Breathe out all the way while squeezing in. Now hold this "vise" tightly when you inhale. As your *lower pear* expands, you will be exercising your diaphragm muscle. Your fingers and thumbs will be slowly forced open. Do this six to ten times, with a 4-count inhale and a 6-to-8-count exhale. Take a regular breath in between each squeeze to give yourself a rest, to feel the flush of blood to this area, and to note any other changes. Any dizziness suggests a low tolerance for energy. If dizzy, wait 30–60 seconds before doing more in order to give your body a chance to absorb the excess energy.

When practiced regularly over time, this exercise can improve your diaphragmatic action and increase your lung volume. For more advanced techniques to quickly and easily achieve optimal breathing, visit www.Breathing.com.

The 70/30 Ratio

No breathing pattern is static, but experience has shown that a good pattern should have a strong tendency toward this 70/30 ratio, due to the sufficient support needed by one's internal core—also known as the *dan tien*, the *hara*, or the internal foundation—which includes the diaphragm.

This 70/30 ratio may change dramatically—even to its opposite of 30/70—when the system encounters extreme degrees of stress or distress. By consciously directing your breath, you can gently and consciously bring your breathing back to the 70/30 balance to better manage and recover from the distress.

In the *#176 Breathing Development Fundamentals* program [see Resources], this area is called "the bottom of the pear." We also liken it to the "basement" of an office building, with the "building" being the lungs, and the "elevator" being the diaphragm, which rises and descends with the breath. ◼

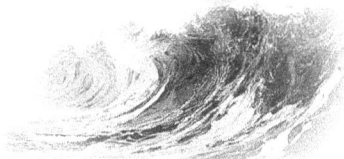

What's a Breath-Work Seminar?

Breathing isn't work—it's automatic—right? So, why attend a Breath-Work Seminar? This seminar focuses on the most important, yet most neglected, activity you do to provide yourself with life and vitality! At the Integral Breathwork Seminars, we measure, assess, and work on improving your breathing function. Then we lie down for a one-hour breathing session that will likely be one of the most life-changing experiences of your life, so far!

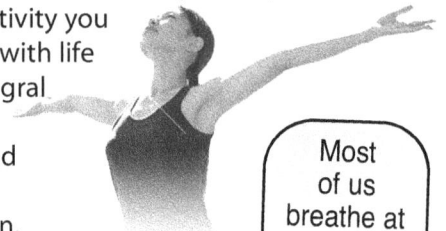

> Most of us breathe at **only 10%** of our full capacity!

After the breathwork session, it's hard to describe how you feel, but some have tried. Here are some actual words that participants have used:

Happy... Relieved... Alive & free... Expanded... I feel like myself again!... Peaceful... Warm & tingly... Strong... Connected to life... Radiant... Aerated!... Drained & refilled... Comfortable... Effervescent... Clearer... More present... Phenomenal!

After a lifetime of studying and sharing about the breath and working with many of the world's experts in this field. After having taught this seminar 100 times, I guarantee that you will benefit and learn life-giving tools, or your money back!

Is this seminar for those with breathing dysfunctions? Absolutely! You will improve significantly and learn how to keep getting better. Is this work for those who feel their breathing is fine, but "feel stuck" in other ways? YES, this work will get you unstuck and give you tools to adjust to, and go with, all of your stressors. You'll LOVE this seminar!

I hope to see you in either Billings or Livingston, from 12:30 to 5:30 pm . Call or e-mail me with any questions you may have... Be sure to pre-register, because space is limited, and I can send you our 6-page Information & Registration Packet.

BODYWORKERS! To bring your CEU credits to six hours, spend an additional hour learning how to incorporate more Breathwork into your Bodywork—it's the perfect marriage! This session continues at the end of the seminar. (Bring a portable table.) ∎

—Denis Ouellette, International Seminar Leader

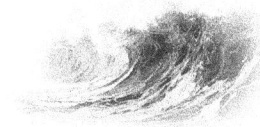

Typical Seminar Agenda

1) INTRODUCTIONS
Who you are? Where are you from? What do you do? What do you want to get out of this seminar?

2) MEASUREMENTS
a) Partner observations: *Chest or belly breather? Neck & shoulder movement during inhale?*
b) Tape measurement, upper chest
c) Do all seven Self-Test Assessments (if time), then review, with ramifications.

3) MEDITATION (with ocean soundtrack)
a) Ocean of energy surrounds you
b) Experiment with deep belly breathing
c) Mentally scan body for blocked energy
d) Send breath and energy to blocked area
e) Use hands to deliver energy

BREAK: E-3 LIVE (Chlorophyll) DRINKS

4) PHYSIOLOGY AND EXERCISES
a) Leaning forward to activate kidney area (diaphragm - chest vs. belly breathing)
b) "Birdie Breath" rapid, shallow, nasal
c) "Fire Breath" *dan tien* breathing
d) "Relaxation Breath" 4-in, 8-out count
e) Paul von Blockmann's Exercises (handout)
f) Squeeze and Breathe (Mike White) (handout)

BREAK: DO STRAPPING TECHNIQUE
Note: Not taught in this book. Effective tool for chest and rib expansion during inhale. See instructions and videos in Mike White's *Optimal Breathing Self-Mastery Kit* at: Breathing.com/pages/the-optimal-breathing-kit

COMMERCIALS: BOOK, CD, E3LIVE, ETC.

5) AUTONOMIC NERVOUS SYSTEM
Are You Stuck In Fight or Flight?
a) Trauma and Stress Ramifications
b) Primitive Brain vs. Prefrontal Cortex

6) BREATHWORK COACHING
a) The Pear, the Cone & the Wave
b) Belly Breathing = entire lower torso
c) Exhale: Throat relaxed, jaw open
d) Total surrender on the exhale
e) Circular Breathing (demo of breathing CD)
f) What to Do • What to Expect (Read verbatim.)

FINAL BREAK (Rest room, Pads & blankets setup)

7) GOAL SETTING (see handout)

8) BREATHWORK SESSION
20 mins. = Use Level One of *Healing Art of Conscious Breathing* CD
40 mins. = Music for Stages Two & Three

9) FRUIT & NUT FEAST WITH DISCUSSION CIRCLE & SEALING
Ask everyone how they feel right now. Ask for volunteers for more lengthy descriptions of their sessions. The food and discussion will help to ground them and end the session. If someone is still deeply processing, have a facilitator stay with them until finished. For *Sealing and Grounding Exercises,* see Katherine the Healer (Chapter 19).

10) FOLLOW UP SHEETS & EVALUATION SHEETS (Chapter 31)

Breathwork Facilitator Coaching:

1) **FACILITATORS:** You're not their therapist, only a facilitator. You're there to see to their comfort. Be non-directive and non-invasive.

2) This is not talk therapy, and you can't see what's going on with them. ***Use your intuition.*** Lean in and give them a good breathing pattern to follow. Coach them through any stuck breathing patterns. Get their belly moving (diaphragmatic breathing).

   Questions should be brief, such as: "Are you cold, hot, or good?" "Do you need a sip of water?" Would a little massage on your hands be helpful?" Never ask, "What's going on with you right now?" This leads to talking that can take them out of their session.

   Read the instructions given by Cochise and Katherine the Healer and all the contributors here. There are breathworker trainings available, and certifications, some of them quite lengthy and expensive. I agree with Dan Brulé in this regard, that breathwork should be mostly freely given and freely received. It is a gift and **the Holy Spirit does the work**. That being said, it is a psychotherapist's tool as well, especially for more difficult situations (i.e., trauma victims, etc.).

3) I choose facilitators based on previous therapy experience. I usually pay them $40 or, if it's a weekend training, we meet on Friday evening for instructions and THEIR session.

4) **SEMINAR TIMING.** I've done this seminar in 4, 5 and 6 hours. In the 4-hour, it's mainly about the breathwork session. In the 5-hour, you can't do all 7 of Mike White's breathing-test measurements, just the first 3 or 4, and you need to cut down on a lot of discussion. In the 6-hour, you have time for everything—and it goes by FAST!

5) More specific training and participant handouts are located throughout the book.

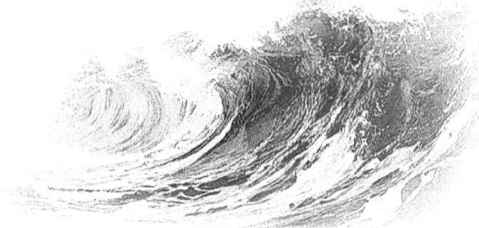

— Seminar Schedule —
12:30 – 6:30 pm

12:30 — Registration & Introductions

1:00 — Optimal Breathing Assessments & Measurements

1:45 — Physiology & Psychology of Breathwork; Q & A

2:30 — Breathwork Exercises & Demonstrations

3:00 — Goal Setting & Prep

3:30 — Group Breathwork Session

5:00 — Sharing & Discussion, with Fruit & Nut Feast, Short Break

5:30 — Bodyworks for Breathworkers

6:30 — Closing

— What to Bring —

1. A moderately empty stomach. Breathwork is more effective without a full stomach. A light pre-noon lunch or brunch will be fine. (Snack foods will be available.)

2. A mat or foam pad to lie on and a quilt or blanket to cover yourself. (The breathwork is done lying on the floor.)

3. A bath towel, to be rolled in a specific way for a headrest & neck roll (see picture).

4. Pad of paper and pen. You may want to take notes during the brief lectures; however, the book has everything in it.

5. A "squirt-bottle" of drinking water.

6. Please bring some fruit or nuts to share for our feast, which we will enjoy while integrating and discussing our experiences.

7. **Bodyworkers:** Bring portable massage table.

— Follow Up —

What To Do After the Seminar

- Take the next day off. Drink plenty of water. Eat lightly.

- It may take a day or two for all the oxygenation and detoxing to move through your body.

- If cleansing is new for you, or if you're on medications, your cells can release excess toxins or chemicals, which can move into your bloodstream. Rest. Drink liquids. Get a massage.

- Write in your journal. Describing your experiences helps to ground and integrate them. What is different now? Set new goals for yourself...

- If emotional and/or psychological issues come up, call your facilitator, or talk it through with a trusted friend or counselor.

Doing More Breathwork at Home

- Practice full-torso breathing always!

- Keep improving your breathing and keep using the newly opened breathing places in your body.

- Do the Von Boeckmann and the Squeeze & Breathe exercises.

- Do 20-minute "maintenance breathing" using the pattern on the CD. Gradually increase lengths and levels.

- The major cleansing and dramatic energy releases usually happen during guided sessions and at the seminars. In your own breathwork, if the movement of energy gets too intense, simply slow down your breathing, gently end your session, and rest. Find a breathing buddy and trade sessions.

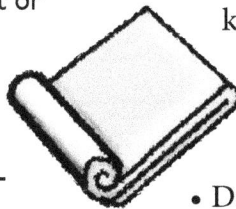

Integral Breathwork™ Seminars
— REGISTRATION FORM —

☐ **Seminar Fee:** *Pre-registered* **$**_____ • *add* **$5** *at door*
☐ **Bring-a-Friend!** *Two for* **$**_____ • *add* **$5** *at door*
☐ **Seminar Repeats:** **$25 off**

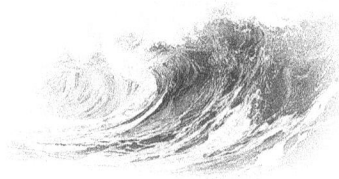

Seminar Date: _____ **Location:** _____

Name _____ **Date of Birth** _____

Address _____

City/State/Zip _____

Phone _____ **E-Mail** _____

PRINT CLEARLY: for notification of upcoming seminars.

For your Breathwork safety, please list any health conditions or concerns (mental, emotional or physical) you now have and any therapies you are currently pursuing. Please list any past surgical operations and current medications.

_____
_____
_____
_____

Please describe your level of experience with Breathwork.

_____
_____
_____

Acknowledgment of Responsibility and Liability Release

I am reserving my Breathwork Seminar space through payment with this form.

I accept full personal responsibility for my physical, emotional and mental well-being. I acknowledge that the leaders make no medical claims whatsoever. I will hold the seminar leaders and their assistants, and the premises, harmless for any outcome as a result of my experiences with this seminar. I sign that I am free from any serious condition that would counter-indicate my participation in this seminar. I will seek out the appropriate therapeutic and/or medical assistance when and as needed.

Your Signature: _____ **Date:** _____

Sponsored by Integral Breathwork™ Seminars

To secure your place at the seminar, please make your check payable to: _____ and mail to: _____

Evaluation • **Integral Breathwork™ Seminars**

Your Name *(optional)* _____ Phone number: _____

Date & Location of Seminar Attended: ____/____/____ _____

1. What were the strengths of the seminar?

_____
_____
_____
_____

2. What could we do better?

_____
_____
_____
_____

3. We plan to offer this seminar periodically in your area. Would you come again?

_____

4. Would you recommend this seminar to a friend?

_____

5. Would you be interested in doing private Breathwork sessions?

_____

6. Would you be interested in private, in-depth physiological Optimal Breathing development?

_____

7. Would you be interested in training as an Integral Breathwork practitioner?

_____

8. Any other comments?

_____
_____

Thank you for joining us! Keep breathing!

Mail to _____

OUR NERVOUS SYSTEMS

CENTRAL NERVOUS SYSTEM
Conscious and Voluntary

↓

**Brain and spinal cord sensory
and motor impulses**

Conditions & Disorders Associated with Overactive Sympathetic Tone (*Stuck-in-Fight or Flight*)

*Most diseases are either caused or made worse by poor breathing,
oxygen starvation, and/or overactive sympathetic tone.*

anxiety or panic attacks	constipation or diarrhea	immune deficiency
allergies	depression	irregular heartbeat
arthritis	digestion problems	irritability
asthma	drug addiction	nightmares or night sweats
back pain	eating disorders	pneumonia
bronchitis	emphysema	sleep apnea or sleep problems
candida, Epstein-Barr	headaches or migraines	snoring
chronic fatigue	high blood pressure	thyroid problems
chronic pain	hyperventilation	weight issues
concentration/memory problems	infertility and impotence	

*Breathing
Affects Both*

CONSCIOUS MIND

External Stimuli

**Over-attention
to negative thoughts,
feelings, and images**
(fears, worries)

UNCONSCIOUS MIND

Internal Stimuli

**Dream recall, altered
states of consciousness**
(unresolved patterns,
internalized trauma)

AUTONOMIC NERVOUS SYSTEM
Unconscious and Involuntary

SYMPATHETIC NERVOUS SYSTEM

Emergency Mode: *"Fight-or-Flight"*

- Increases blood flow to the heart, primitive brain, and large muscles
- Releases adrenaline
- Increases heart rate and blood pressure
- Slows or stops immune system and digestion

IMBALANCES:

- High blood pressure
- Digestive disorders
- Poor circulation (cold hands & feet)
- Irregular heartbeat
- Migraines, neck and back pain
- Peptic ulcers
- Anxiety or panic disorders

(see list opposite page)

Characterized by high-chest rapid breathing and/or holding the breath

PARASYMPATHETIC NERVOUS SYSTEM

"Rest, Digest & Heal"

- Decreases heart rate and blood pressure
- Increases blood flow to high brain, digestive organs, and skin
- Activates immune system

IMBALANCES:

- Low blood pressure
- Poor appetite, apathy
- Non-responsiveness to stress or emergency

Characterized by slower diaphragmatic (belly) breathing

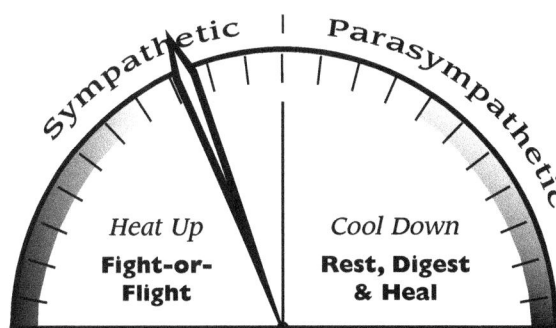

Sympathetic | Parasympathetic

Heat Up
Fight-or-Flight

Cool Down
Rest, Digest & Heal

Autonomic Nervous System

Body, Mind, Emotions, and Environment Are Stimulators

Toxicity, negative thoughts, stress, and anxiety trigger overactive sympathetic.
Deep, relaxed diaphragmatic breathing calms sympathetic and activates parasympathetic.

OUR NERVOUS SYSTEMS

CENTRAL NERVOUS SYSTEM
Brain to Nerves to Muscles
**Conscious breathing accesses autonomic system via central nervous system
to repair and calm sympathetic autonomic responses**

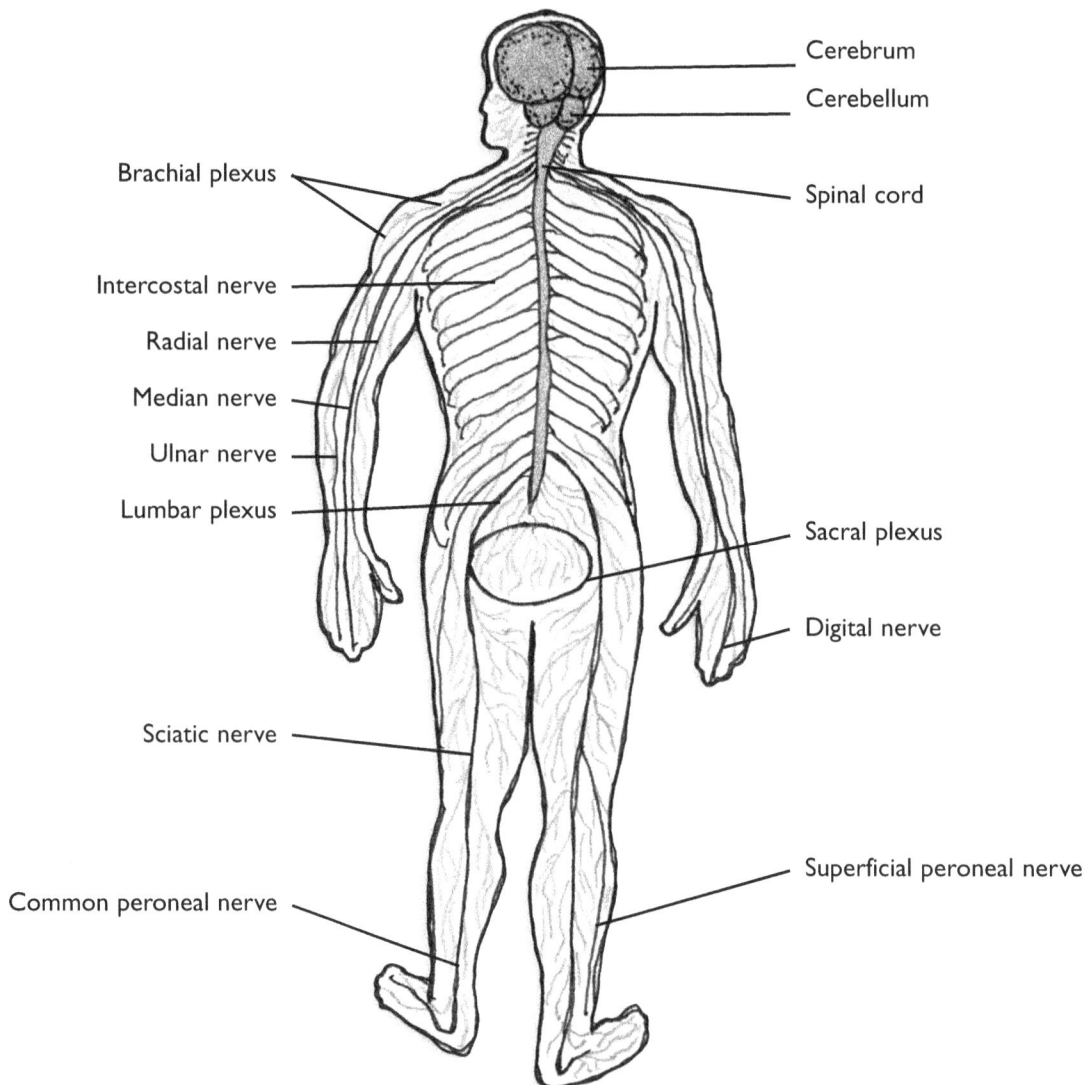

Cerebrum
Cerebellum

Brachial plexus

Spinal cord

Intercostal nerve

Radial nerve

Median nerve

Ulnar nerve

Lumbar plexus

Sacral plexus

Digital nerve

Sciatic nerve

Superficial peroneal nerve

Common peroneal nerve

The brain can be subdivided into several distinct regions: The **cerebral hemispheres** form the largest part of the brain, occupying the anterior and middle area of the skull and extending backwards. Within these is the **diencephalon**, which forms the central core of the brain and includes the thalamus, hypothalamus, epithalamus, and subthalamus. The **midbrain** is located at the junction of the middle and posterior cranial fossae. The **pons** connects one cerebral hemisphere with its opposite cerebellar hemisphere. The **medulla oblongata** is continuous with the spinal cord and is responsible for automatic control of the respiratory and cardiovascular systems. The **cerebellum** overlies the pons and medulla. It is mainly concerned with motor functions that regulate muscle tone, coordination, and posture.

AUTONOMIC NERVOUS SYSTEM
Internal Organ and System Function
Access to unconscious autonomic system is possible through conscious breathing via the central nervous system

SYMPATHETIC
"Fight-or-Flight"

PARASYMPATHETIC
"Rest, Digest & Heal"

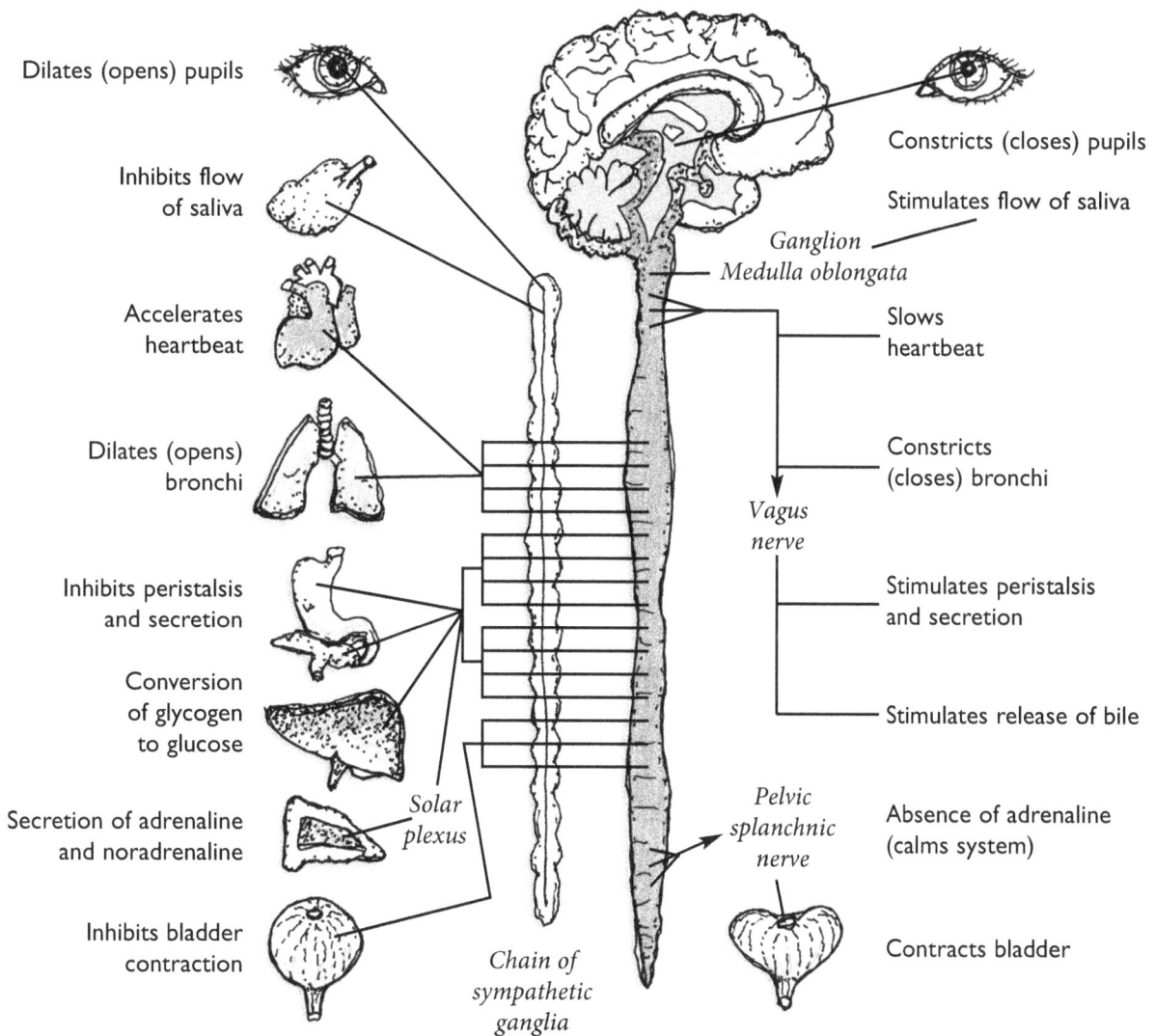

Dilates (opens) pupils

Inhibits flow of saliva

Accelerates heartbeat

Dilates (opens) bronchi

Inhibits peristalsis and secretion

Conversion of glycogen to glucose

Secretion of adrenaline and noradrenaline

Inhibits bladder contraction

Solar plexus

Chain of sympathetic ganglia

Constricts (closes) pupils

Stimulates flow of saliva

Ganglion
Medulla oblongata

Slows heartbeat

Constricts (closes) bronchi

Vagus nerve

Stimulates peristalsis and secretion

Stimulates release of bile

Pelvic splanchnic nerve

Absence of adrenaline (calms system)

Contracts bladder

Nerves all along the mid-spine (L2 to T1) contain the **sympathetic stimulators**. The vagus nerve is the main **parasympathetic stimulator** to most of the body's organs (from lungs, heart, and liver, to stomach, kidneys, and ascending and transverse colon). The vagus nerve is located at the medulla where the spine attaches to the skull (above C1). The pelvic splanchnic nerve (at S2–4) is the parasympathetic stimulator for the bladder, prostate, urethra, reproductive organs, and descending colon. **Breathwork can stimulate either** the sympathetic (hyperventilation) or the parasympathetic (de-stressing breathing), depending on the breathing pattern's rapidity, localization, intent, length of inhalation vs. exhalation, and other factors.

WHAT TO DO

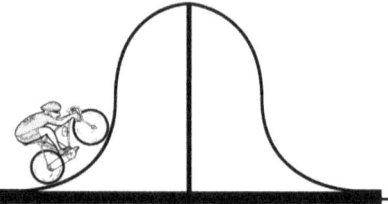

STAGE ONE =

Drink some water and use the restroom. *Water in—water out!*
Lie down with a small, neck support (chin slightly upward).
Lay a small, pillow (or towel) along the spine at the mid-back (optional),
   as this opens the chest and allows the shoulders to fall back.
Cover your body halfway with a blanket.
No jewelry or glasses. Loosen tight belt and/or clothes (including bras).
Have water handy (squirt bottle).

Begin full, smooth, circular connected breathing.
No holding between inhales or exhales.
In-and-out breathing through the mouth or nose is OK at this point.
Fill the abdominal area, then the rib cage, then the upper lungs.
Relax and let go on the exhale.
Surrender to gravity on the exhale.
Do not push the air out or hold it back.
Relax the jaw and the tongue; open the throat.
Cover yourself more or less, as needed.
Have sips of water as needed.
Follow the breathing pattern on the CD or set by the facilitator.

> Please read from left, across the page, to right.
> **STAGE ONE** is *"First Gear - Uphill,"* etc.

STAGE TWO =

Stay with the breathing.
Allow all physical sensations to pass through you.
Feel free to experience your emotions.
Remember to relax and surrender on the exhale.
Raise your hand if you need any assistance.
You'll soon be over the hump—the rest is easy street.
Enjoy the music.

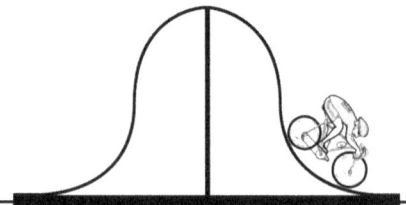

STAGE THREE =

Continue to breathe, but you can ease up on it.
Breathing through your nose (in and out) is better at this point.
Enjoy how your body and energy levels feel.
Enjoy your new breathing freedom.
Relax until all sensations have subsided, then
   raise your knees and/or roll over on your side.

WHAT TO EXPECT

First Gear - Uphill (approx. 20 minutes)

Some effort is required to achieve a good breathing pattern.
Stay with it; work with it.
You're oxygenating your body and releasing toxins.
You're breaking through self-limiting mental and emotional patterns.
You're moving new life and energy through.

As your nervous system balances itself and your body processes and self-cleanses,
    you may experience some of these sensations:
        Dry mouth (if mouth breathing, OK to take sips of water).
        Tingling or numbness in parts of your body,
          most often in the hands, feet or mouth areas.
        Body temperature shifts, cold or hot (sweating).
        Ringing or buzzing frequencies in the ears.
        Heaviness or drowsiness (toxin release).
        Waves of emotion (OK to feel them).
        Waves of energy (fun to feel them).
        Breath release (expansion).

Second Gear - the Peak (approx. 20 minutes)

If muscle stiffness or cramping (tetany) occurs, or any uncomfortability, relax on and
    slow down the exhale, switch to nose/nose breathing, make sure you're doing
    diaphragmatic *(parasympathetic)* breathing, and allow all sensations to pass.
They will soon subside. Ask for assistance when needed.
If memory recall or extrasensory experiences occur, it works well to
    experience them, honor them, and let them pass.
Surrender to and trust the higher intelligence of this healing process.
Always return to your breath as your trusted vehicle.

Third Gear - Home Stretch (approx. 20 minutes)

A sense of peace, calm, and renewed energy.
Mental and emotional clarity.
Opened and expanded breathing.
A stress-free physical body.

Ample time will be given for integration and completion of your experience.
We follow the breathwork session with a fruit feast, discussion circle, and
    grounding and sealing exercises. ▪

GOAL SETTING

[After the *What To Do—What To Expect* handout (see previous pages) is read aloud verbatim, a co-counseling process is done in pairs immediately before lying down for the one-hour breathwork session. Play some soft music. I like one with an ocean track on it for some white noise to help prevent overhearing. The leader instructs the participants to set up their blankets and bolsters alongside their partner's and to get everything ready for their sessions (water bottles handy, etc.). Then the leader begins as follows:]

Because breathwork can go off in so many directions, it's always good to set some goals for your session beforehand. This is an 8-minute process. Each of you will have one minute to talk about each of the four areas—physical, mental, emotional, and memories. Partners will take turns sharing in each of these areas. First, sit up and face your partner. Introduce yourselves to each other. Now decide who will talk first and who will listen. If you're both comfortable with it, a little physical contact is good—knees, hands, or whatever. We'll start by giving each other some assurances. You'll repeat these statements after me:

"I assure you of complete safety and confidentiality. / I promise I won't ever repeat what you say either to you or to anyone else. / In fact, I'm probably going to forget the whole thing. / This is for your benefit only. / I'm not here to give you any advice, just to listen with an open heart."

Now your partner gives these same assurances.

[Leader restates the above assurances for the partners to repeat.]

We'll use a chime to alert you when it's time to switch partners.

ONE — The Physical

OK, switch back to the first partner, and talk for one minute about your physical concerns. Where are your chronic pains? Your old injuries? Where in your body do you need healing? What are you ready to let go of today? Where do you want to get some good energy flowing? OK, for one minute, go ahead.

[Sound the chime to start. At 50 seconds, say "10 seconds" to warn people to finish. Sound the chime at 60 seconds.]

Switch partners and talk about your physical concerns for one minute. Go.

[Sound the chime to start. At 50 seconds, say "10 seconds" to warn people to finish. Sound the chime at 60 seconds.]

TWO — The Mental

Next we do the mental issues. Here, you discuss stuck negative mental thoughts or attitudes and repeating patterns—broken records—that you really feel tired of and done with. It could be negative attitudes about life, about money, a family member, your boss, or anything. OK, for one minute, go.

[Sound the chime to start. At 50 seconds, say "10 seconds" to warn people to finish. Sound the chime at 60 seconds.]

OK, switch partners and talk about stuck mental patterns you are ready to let go of. One minute.

[Sound the chime to start. At 50 seconds, say "10 seconds" to warn people to finish. Sound the chime at 60 seconds.]

THREE — The Emotional

Now, for the emotions. Some say all our emotions tend to boil down to the basic four: mad, sad, glad, or scared. So let's focus on mad, sad, or scared. What are you angry about? What are you unhappy about? And what are you afraid of? OK, let's do one minute on mad, sad, or scared. Begin.

[Sound the chime to start. At 50 seconds, say "10 seconds" to warn people to finish. Sound the chime at 60 seconds.]

Now switch partners and talk about mad, sad, or scared.

[Sound the chime to start. At 50 seconds, say "10 seconds" to warn people to finish. Sound the chime at 60 seconds.]

FOUR — The Memories

OK, the last segment is the memories. Here we can go back five minutes, five hours, five days, or to five or fifty years ago. It doesn't matter. Just talk about whatever comes into your mind as a memory you'd like to have the healing breath pass through today. One minute. Go.

[Sound the chime to start. At 50 seconds, say "10 seconds" to warn people to finish. Sound the chime at 60 seconds.]

Now switch partners and talk about your memories.

[Sound the chime to start. At 50 seconds, say "10 seconds" to warn people to finish. Sound the chime at 60 seconds.]

Conclusion

Thank your partner and feel free to give them a hug. OK, now take a little time to separate out and get into your own space. Stay sitting up for a little while longer, and reflect briefly on everything you said. Now surrender it. It's like letting a toy boat go sailing on a pond. All or none of these goals may actually be achieved today. Changes may occur in the days ahead. Now that you've set the sail, you can let it go and surrender to the healing process and the higher intelligence guiding it.

Now you're ready for your breathwork sessions. You can lie down, make yourselves comfortable, and begin the breathing process.

We'll turn on the breathing pattern for the first few minutes. Follow it if it works for you. If it feels too fast or too much, breathe at a rhythm and volume that feels right for you. We're here to assist you if you need anything.

[If tears come up during the verbal processing, as they often will—because people don't often get the chance to speak and be listened to this intimately or safely—the facilitators can go around with tissues.

Before lying down, partners may need to spread out their mats and blankets a little to allow the facilitators to pass freely around the participants.

Announce that people may use the restroom one more time before the breathwork begins.]

SEVEN CHAKRAS & ASSOCIATIONS

CHAKRA *Location*	GLAND/ORGAN *Systems & Areas*	COLOR Musical Note *Bija Mantra*	Associations
CROWN *Top of the head, extending upward*	PINEAL *Brain & nervous system, skin*	YELLOW B *Ah*	Universal consciousness, illumination, wisdom & education, direction & intuition
THIRD-EYE *Center of forehead*	PITUITARY *Endocrine system, sinuses, eyes, ears & nose*	GREEN A *Om*	Healing, abundance, truth, the arts, concentration, clairvoyance, dreams, Christ consciousness
THROAT *At the throat*	THYROID *Respiratory/lungs, metabolism, larynx, throat & mouth*	BLUE G *Ham*	Protection, perfection, faith, the will of God, communication, creativity & self-expression
HEART *Center of chest*	THYMUS *Heart & circulatory, upper back, shoulders & arms*	PINK F *Yam*	Adoration & devotion, ability to give & receive unconditional love
SOLAR PLEXUS *Above the navel*	PANCREAS *Stomach/spleen, small intestines, liver/gall bladder, digestion, middle back*	PURPLE & GOLD E *Ram*	Service to others, acceptance, emotional & personal power
SEAT-OF-THE-SOUL or SACRAL *Below the navel*	GONADS *Reproductive, kidneys, bladder & prostate, assimilation, lower back & hips*	VIOLET D *Vam*	Mercy & forgiveness, sexuality & desires, general health of the lower body
BASE or ROOT *Base of the Spine*	ADRENALS *Bladder, colon, skeletal & spine, lymph & immune, elimination, legs*	WHITE C *Lam*	Anchoring of the four lower bodies, security & money, connection with earth, font of kundalini

This is a compilation from several of the world's chakra systems to illustrate and clarify the text. The musical notes and *bija* mantras (syllables that encapsulate the essence of the chakra) may be sounded in conjunction with the Essene Rebirth and other healing work. Many systems portray the chakra colors along the rainbow spectrum, starting with red at the base chakra and ending with violet at the crown. I am using the chakra colors as taught in the esoteric school of the Theosophical Society, which continues its legacy today as the Teachings of the Ascended Masters. In their view, the color scheme listed here portrays the purified etheric hues of the chakras and represents their ultimate purpose as indicated in the associations. I have added these colors for correct visualization during the Essene Rebirth section in Part Two. For beautiful illustrations of the chakras in this system by artist Marius Michael-George, visit www.MariusFineArt.com.

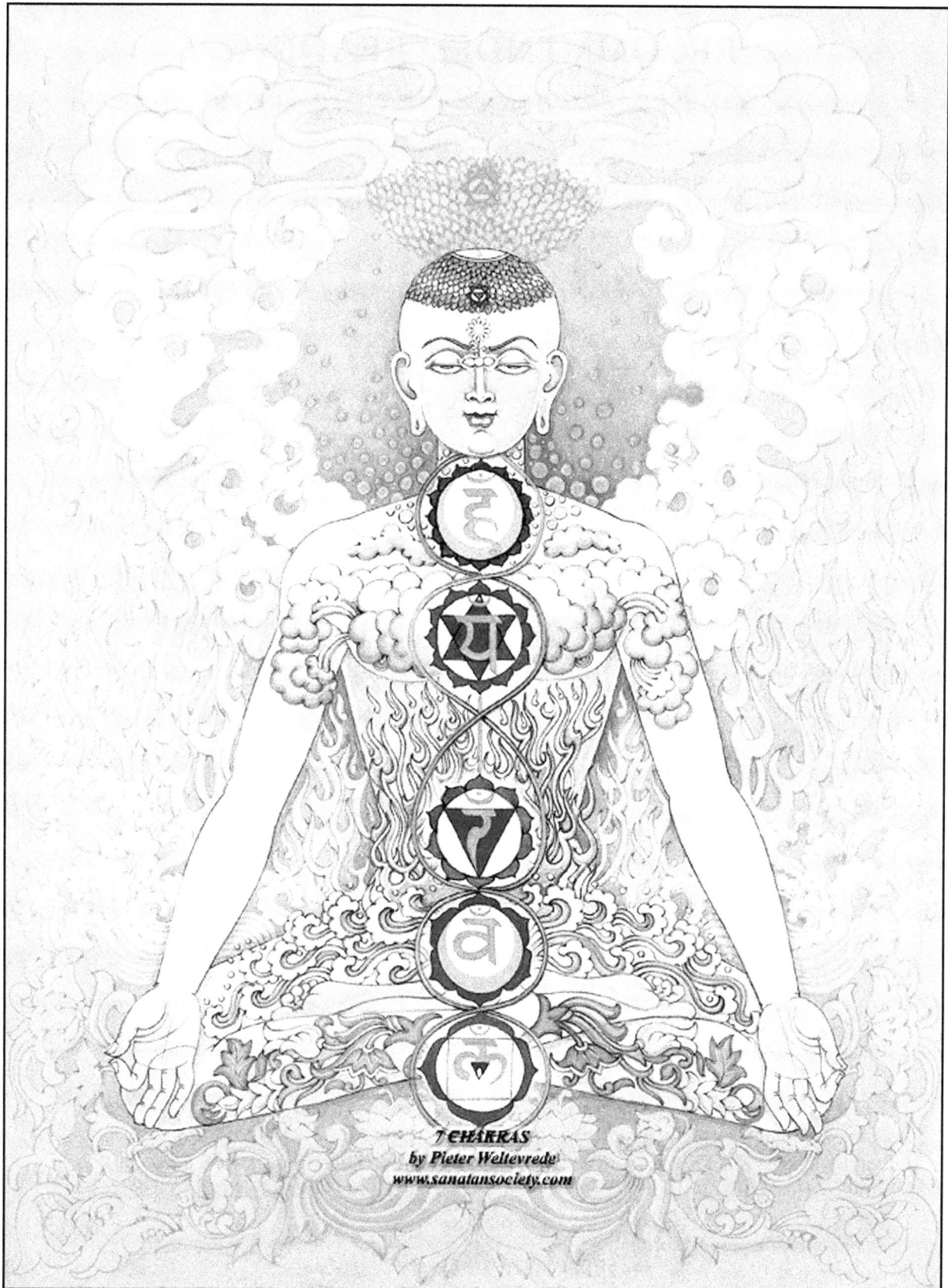

Illustration of the seven chakras, showing the Sanskrit inscription for the *bija* mantra within each chakra, the caduceus interplay (winged rod with snakes intertwined) of the kundalini, and the progression of the four elements. Courtesy of Pieter Weltevrede and www.SanatanSociety.com.

RECOMMENDED READING
for Breathwork & Healing Work

The Art of Conscious Breathing:
Selected Articles (available soon);
and *Chi Kung: A Brief Introduction to Chinese*
Medical Breathing Exercises
Dan Brulé
Visit www.BreathMastery.com

Chakra Breathing: Breath as Pathway to
Energy, Harmony and Self-Healing
Helmut G. Sieczka

Chi Gung: Harnessing the Power of the
Universe (Shambhala Publications)
Daniel P. Reid

Conscious Breathing: How Shamanic
Breathwork Can Transform Your Life; and
Soul Therapy
Joy Manné, PhD
Visit www.i-breathe.com

Conscious Healing: Book One
on the Regenetics Method
Sol Luckman

Free Your Breath, Free Your Life: How
Conscious Breathing Can Relieve Stress,
Increase Vitality, and Help You Live
More Fully
Dennis Lewis

Hara: The Vital Center of Man
Karlfried Graf Dürckheim

The Healing Breath: A Journal of Breathwork
Practice, Psychology, and Spirituality
Edited by Joy Manné, PhD
Visit www.HealingBreathJournal.org

The Hidden Messages in Water;
The Message of Water, Vols. 1 & 2; and
The Power of Water (DVD/VHS)
Dr. Masaru Emoto

Kundalini, Evolution and Enlightenment
Edited by John White

The Kundalini Experience:
Psychosis or Transcendence?
Lee Sanella, MD

The Power of Emotion
Michael Sky

The Secret Power of Music: The
Transformation of Self and Society
Through Musical Energy
David Tame

Secrets of Optimal Natural Breathing; and
Building Healthy Lungs Naturally
Michael Grant White
Visit www.Breathing.com

The Tao of Health, Sex & Longevity, A
Modern Practical Guide to the Ancient Way
(Simon & Schuster)
Daniel P. Reid
Visit www.DanielReid.org

The Water Puzzle and the Hexagonal Key:
Scientific Evidence of Hexagonal Water and Its
Positive Influence on Health
Dr. Mu Shik Jhon

NOTE: For an extensive reading list
(43 pages) see *An Annotated Book List*
for Breathwork Training, compiled by
Catherine Dowling and Joy Manné in
The Healing Breath, Vol. 3, No. 2.
Visit www.HealingBreathJournal.org

SUGGESTED MUSIC
for Breathwork & Healing Work

John Barry: Soundtrack, *Somewhere in Time, Main Theme*	*emotional*
Rachmaninoff: *Rhapsody on a Theme of Paganini*	*emotional*
Samuel Barber: *Adagio for Strings, Opus 11*	*moving*
J.S. Bach: *Air on the G String*	*majestic*
Jerry Goldsmith: Soundtrack, *First Knight*, "Camelot Lives"	*uplifting*
Pietro Mascagni: Intermezzo, *Cavalleria Rusticana*	*profound*
John Rutter: *Requiem*, "Pie Jesu"	*peaceful*
W.A. Mozart: *Ave Verum Corpus*	*soulful*
W.A. Mozart: *Hostias, Requiem in D Minor*	*holy*
Johannes Brahms: *Wie Lieblich Sind Deine Wohnungen*	*holy*
Celine Dion (artist): *Brahm's Lullaby* (Album: *Miracle*)	*inner child reunion*
Edward Elgar: *Nimrod, Enigma Variations*	*settling*
Antonin Dvorak: *New World Symphony, No. 9, Largo*	*relieving*
Vaughan Williams: *Lark Ascending*	*emerging*
Album, Laurel Emryss: *Welcome to Earthaven*	*ethereal, peaceful*

Breathwork heightens the acuity of the senses and places the participant in a vulnerable, receptive state. The music being played during breathwork influences the client in very emotional and physical ways. It's as though the music is being played right through them, so it is of paramount importance that the musical choices be of a quality that will complement this process and lead them in the direction of healing and peace. David Tame, author of *The Secret Power of Music* [see Recommended Reading], and others have shown that the syncopated beat in much of today's music (rock, rap, pop, jazz) has a detrimental effect on people's vitality, throwing off the natural rhythms of the body. Some believe this beat causes an energy-dissipating (counterclockwise) spin of the chakras. A syncopated beat is characterized by the displacement of the regular metrical accent of the 4/4 time. Rather than coming in on the first beat (the downbeat), the accent is asymmetrically placed on the third beat, as in "one, two, THREE, four." Listen for it, and you'll find this rhythm to be ubiquitous in today's culture. We may enjoy these types of music for recreation, but I recommend they be avoided for healing work.

Today's market is flooded with new-age music titles. After a thorough search, I find that much of this music does not rise to the level of true inspiration and elevation I look for to achieve a therapeutic effect. Some of it contains an underlying syncopation. Other pieces are too sleepy or ethereal. There are certainly notable exceptions within this genre. Additionally, there is some excellent music coming out of the film industry; soundtracks are a prime avenue of expression for some of today's best composers. Soundtracks with cuts I recommend for healing include *Tuck Everlasting, Anna and the King (new version), Band of Brothers, Anastasia, Meet Joe Black,* and *Shakespeare in Love.*

My personal favorites remain with the timeless classics and with the world's best sacred, choral and orchestral music, while including some of this century's great composers. Above is the music list I employ during our breathwork sessions, in specific sequence. I've included emotional keywords to illustrate the feeling expressed by each piece. Many of these will often have personal significance for the listeners. (We usually start the session with a few minutes of the breathing-pattern CD. See Resources.) This series invariably brings good results and wonderful benefits for the client. All of these titles can be had from the iTunes store.

When our breathwork sessions are winding down and we transition to reemergence, our fruit feast, discussion circle, grounding and sealing, I invariably use *Welcome to Earthaven* by Laurel Emryss (entire CD) because of the "Elysian-fields," parasympathetic calm this album evokes. ▨

The Healing Art of Conscious Breathing
CD User's Guide

In 2001, I was doing a lot of breathwork and self-esteem work and attending workshops with the pioneers of breathwork, Bob Mandel and Leonard Orr. The one thing missing, it seemed to me, was a tool breathworkers could give their clients to continue their work at home. Even with my own experience in breathwork, I wanted a tool I could use for myself. I remembered reading about breathing and resonances in Itzhak Bentov's book, *Stalking the Wild Pendulum.* With my knowledge of electronics, it dawned on me that connected breathing was similar to a basic sine wave. If the breathing could be recorded correctly, where the inhale and the exhale would follow a sine wave, it would provide that tool. I had no idea where this was leading. I called my sound engineer, Chuck Jopskei, and explained what I needed. This might have seemed comical, but he was intrigued and interested in the challenge.

Our first recording in the studio was quite easy. After two hours of editing, I ended up with a twenty-minute track to take home. What I had was the template for what would become *The Healing Art of Conscious Breathing* CD. The next day, I lay down and started to breathe, synchronizing my breath to the pattern on the CD. I breathed for twenty minutes, then another twenty, and then another. I thought to myself, "Oh my gosh, what did I just create?" If I could get such great results with this CD, maybe anyone could! This was a program people could easily use on their own, along with some basic guidelines on safety and pacing oneself.

But first, back to the studio. The demo had low-level interference from electrical signals that were unknowingly recorded. I knew what was needed. "OK, Chuck, let's do it again. This time, we're making a good one!" This went on for three months. No wonder breathing is so difficult to record. White noise is a monster when it comes to recording low-level sounds, such as breathing, and making them audible and clear. Chuck and I discovered the secrets to recording breathing in the best way possible.

As I was creating this CD, I wanted it to be flexible, with separate tracks, and no instruction mixed in with the breathing tracks. You can program the tracks in any order you choose, or mix them with your favorite music. Many people have told me how helpful the CD has been for them—from stroke victims to people in extreme pain. One stroke victim told me

he fully recovered from the paralysis. Another told me it kept him from going into the hospital. The simplicity of the CD is that it puts you in the driver's seat with your healing work.

Here are some recommendations for using this breathwork CD. Whenever possible, breathe with a partner. If a human isn't available, try your dog or cat. Pets seem to understand the process somehow. Sometimes after breathing on a warm night, I will go outside to get some fresh air. Somehow the cats in the neighborhood sense my cleansed energy and come up to me for some attention. One of my teachers tells the story about a group breathwork session he conducted. His dog came into the room and sat next to one of the participants as he was breathing. The dog was panting, which is a basic connected breath. The participant, whose eyes were closed, followed along, thinking that he was being guided by the teacher. He said afterwards that it was the best breathing session he ever had!

There are disadvantages to breathing alone, especially for beginners, and the main one is the lack of support. When you're breathing by yourself, it's difficult to go deeply into the process. Breathing helps us access the three lower levels of consciousness associated with the delta, theta, and alpha brainwaves. In that sense, it's a regressive process. We go back in mind and body to access and release the trauma of our past experiences. So breathing alone can be like going into a dark cave, not knowing what you'll discover there. It's nice to have a loving friend holding your hand, so to speak.

Be patient with breathwork. Some type-A personalities want to go too fast with their healing. The biggest mistake people make in using the CD is going too fast through the levels. Stay with Level One (the slowest breathing pattern) for quite a while and repeat it until it starts to feel too slow. Breathwork can sneak up on you. As trauma is released, the feelings, tensions, and images that result can at times be overwhelming. That's a good reason to have a partner handy and to start off with shorter sessions at a slower pace. If you develop too much fear and apprehension, you may distance yourself from breathing altogether and lose this all-important healing tool.

The book in your hands is about breathwork, which relates to the element of air, but it's also about healing through the other elements of earth, fire, and water. For me, sometimes air alone just isn't enough. The breath is so powerful in the beginning. It has the ability to awaken the mind and body. As the breath reawakens deep memories, it can trigger feelings of irritability, depression, anxiety, or sadness. It's helpful to remember that these feelings are temporary and part of the purifying process. I do breathwork regularly, and at times stuff just seems to come up on its own. When breathing by itself doesn't clear my energy, I will breathe while soaking in water. If that doesn't work, I will lie by the fireplace and see what that does. At times, I will journal about what I feel is out of order in my life, and I'll write affirmations to counteract my negative thoughts or attitudes. Sometimes I'll go for a walk in nature and let the earth's energies wash over me. One of these elements always works. I haven't taken an aspirin in over ten years. Headaches are rare for me, but when I get one, breathing always helps dissipate them.

Here's why I feel fire and water are so helpful: When you sit in front of fire, your chakras spin and extend out about five feet. When they spin in the fire, they get cleansed, and the emotional weight you're carrying is released into the flames. Water can have a similar effect. Warm water will open your chakras and cleanse them. Cold water will close them and ground you. After I breathe, I find that a warm shower followed by a cold shower will work wonders. After that, I'm ready to take on the world!

Remember to drink plenty of water after breathwork. The body tends to purge itself of toxins when you breathe. This is even more evident when breathing in a tub of water. You may even notice some debris that has been released through the skin settling to the bottom of the tub.

The book you are reading is a great guide and introduction to breathwork and other self-healing techniques. When I read the first edition, it changed my thinking and somehow my vibration. Be patient with your healing. Do it with friends. And honor your process—it's a sacred undertaking. ▪

Sincerely,
John Meneghini

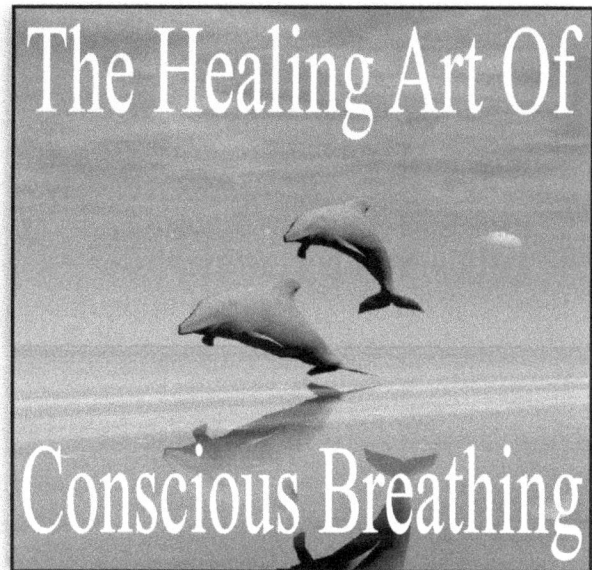

EDITOR'S NOTE: We use this CD with consistently great results in our seminars. We encourage participants to take it home and use it for their personal breathwork. We recommend, as John does, that people pace it slowly, use a partner when available, and start with shorter breathing sessions. We use Level One Breathing for 10 to 20 minutes, depending on the needs of the group. We then play music for the remainder of the session.

I DO TAKE ISSUE with two small items in the Introduction on this CD: Integral Breathwork involves coaching people to adopt sound physiological breathing mechanics before embarking on a session of circular breathing and optimizing oxygen intake.

1) High-chest breathing is recommended... The breathing mechanics outlined in this book explain clearly that diaphragmatic breathing is far more healthful than chest breathing in terms of its effect on the nervous system.

2) Burning incense or a candle is suggested... We would change that to opening a window for some good fresh air!

E3 LIVE: Earth's First Food

Michael Saiber, President of Vision

Amazing Discovery from a Pristine Ancient Lake

There exists in Oregon an almost magical body of water called Upper Klamath Lake. This lake has an exceptionally high mineral concentration created by the volcanic eruption of Mount Mazama that occurred over 7,000 years ago, creating an amazing ecosystem and one of the wonders of the Western world—Crater Lake, which feeds into Upper Klamath Lake. The eruption covered the area with millions of tons of mineral ash. Seventeen streams and rivers deposit mineral-rich volcanic soil from the surrounding 4,000-square-mile basin, making Upper Klamath Lake one of the richest nutrient traps in the world.

It is also one of the few remaining alkaline lakes on the planet. At 4,100 feet elevation, it is surrounded by national forest and timberland, and it is remarkably pure and pristine—*especially* for this day and age.

This pristine lake, literally overflowing with volcanic minerals, harbors one of the world's most amazing nutritional discoveries. About 20 years ago, special fresh-water nutritional plants, referred to as *cyanophyta*, were discovered growing in Upper Klamath Lake. (The area's indigenous peoples have been eating this food for thousands of years.) The powerful form of *cyanophyta* they found is called **Aphanizomenon flos-aquae** (AFA), which literally means "invisible living flower of the water."

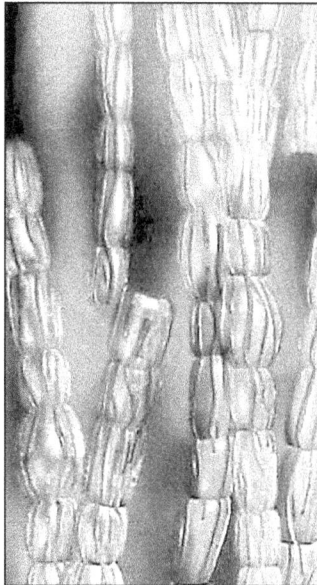

Aphanizomenon flos-aquae
(AFA) "invisible living flower of the water" (magnified)

Why does this matter to you?

Well, for starters, it turns out that *cyanophyta* are collectively responsible for 90% of the earth's oxygen and 80% of its food supply! And while there are tens of thousands of species of these amazing unicellular plants—literally the first plants to make their appearance on planet Earth—not all are edible. Of the edible ones, AFA is in a class by itself. That's the thrilling part about the discovery in Klamath Lake. AFA is now described by natural health experts as **the single most nutritionally complete, health-transforming food on the planet.**

Before you go running to the nearest health food store to look for AFA—*be careful!* Not all AFA is created equally. Much of it is not harvested or handled in a high-quality manner. Plus, most forms of AFA are heavily processed, destroying the vitality and benefit of the original plant.

There is only one company that harvests AFA strictly from the purest region of Upper Klamath Lake and then *exclusively* bottles it fresh. Once it is tested for purity and potency, the pure liquid AFA is then fresh-frozen so there's virtually no degradation or nutrient loss. The company is called Vision, started by a health-conscious Oregon couple in 1995, and they harvest **E3Live™—100% live, fresh-frozen AFA.**

Since it began, Vision has been the ONLY producer in the world of this pure, fresh-frozen aquatic super-food. This unparalleled form of

AFA has rapidly become the health food of choice of many top doctors, world-class athletes, celebrities, and ultimately, *anyone* looking to combat the chemical assault of today's world. People that want to look and feel younger swear by E3Live.

Gabriel Cousens, M.D., is one of the world's foremost holistic medical doctors and the author of *Depression-Free for Life*; *Conscious Eating*; and other books. He's the founder of Tree of Life Rejuvenation Center in Arizona. He says:

As a physician working with thousands of clients, I find that E3Live helps to restore overall biochemical balance by nourishing the body at the cellular level. Our positive response from the use of E3Live has been extraordinary. It's a wonderful and unique source for peak performance of body, mind, and spirit that should be included in any detoxification and rejuvenation program. I take it myself daily.

How the Miracle of E3Live™ Works

So how does E3Live help to instantly replenish your oxygen, nutrition, and vitality levels? For starters, E3Live contains more chlorophyll than any other food in existence—a whopping 160% higher than the next highest food, spirulina, and 3 to 5 times more than wheatgrass.

The amazing fact is that chlorophyll's molecular structure is *almost identical* to that of hemoglobin, which is responsible for carrying oxygenated blood throughout the body.

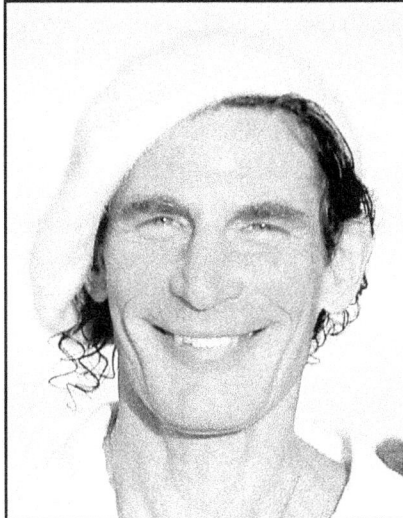

"The E3Live™ liquid algae, Aphanizomenon flos-aquae, is more primitive, and closer to original creation. The beauty of it all is that in the mystical Kabbalistic teaching of Judaism, it is taught that the closer an organism is to the Divine and the beginning of creation, the more powerful it is, and the more energy it has to elevate us spiritually."

—Dr. Gabriel Cousens

So chlorophyll molecules are easily converted into oxygen. This means that AFA's chlorophyll is the central molecule for increasing oxygen availability to your system! Simply put, **there's no food on the planet that can supercharge your body with oxygen faster or more effectively than E3Live!**

Not only that, chlorophyll also detoxifies the body from both internally generated wastes and the external poisons you're bombarded with on a daily basis. And remember—*that's only the beginning.* Years of research by Christian Drapeau, M.A. in Neurology and Neurosurgery, have revealed that AFA contains much more:

✪ Scientists are calling phenylethylamine (PEA) the "molecule of love" because it creates the sense of joy and fulfillment one experiences when in love. PEA is believed to enhance concentration and attention and to quickly elevate your mood.

✪ There have been many scandals about man-made COX-2 drugs and their deadly side effects. But phycocyanin, which is the blue pigment in AFA, is a *safe and natural* COX-2 inhibitor with strong anti-inflammatory properties.

✪ With all of the pollution you face, your immune system needs protection like never before. AFA contains the only known ultra-rare polysaccharide that **stimulates the migration of immune cells in the body.**

✪ The most thrilling news of all is that AFA can actually help you regenerate brand-new healthy cells, completely revitalizing your body! This works because AFA has a unique compound that stimulates stem cell release and migration of your own bone marrow stem cells.

○ E3Live is the highest source of plant protein available and contains all of the amino acids in perfect balance that your body requires. Amino acids are the building blocks of protein. By using E3Live, you are supplying yourself with the best form of plant protein available.

○ It contains over 60 minerals and trace minerals, *in a powerfully chelated form,* so your body can *instantly* absorb them into your cells. With the exception of D and K, *all* vitamins are present in E3Live, giving you the perfect nutrient fuel for your cells. And despite what cereal companies tell you, you don't need to *eat* Vitamin D and K. They're produced naturally by your body under normal conditions.

○ E3Live also contains the much-needed Essential Fatty Acids Omega-3 and Omega-6. And it is one of the highest known natural food sources for beta carotene, a cell regenerator and potent antioxidant—neutralizer of premature aging and damaging free radicals.

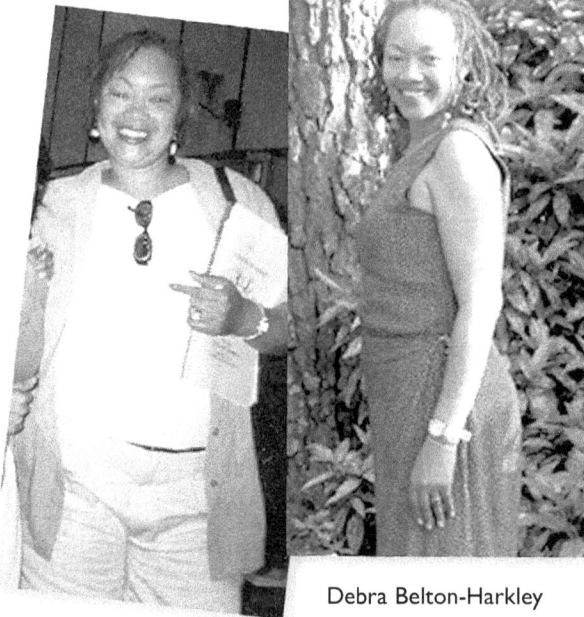

Debra Belton-Harkley

What Do Others Say?

Hundreds of thousands of people worldwide have now enjoyed the amazing, life-changing benefits of E3Live. Here are a few of the many testimonials we've received:

Within 3 days of taking E3Live, I felt better mentally and I did not have the bad cravings for junk food like before. In 2 weeks, I lost 13 lbs. I lost another 27 lbs. in the next two months due to my reduced cravings and had more energy.

—Debra Belton-Harkley

Since I began eating E3Live, I've noticed an unmistakable boost in my energy. I have more stamina and can swim faster for longer periods. My racing times have improved. I can now work out more intensely. Recovery time is dramatically shorter. Bottom line—E3Live makes a big difference in my performance.

—Ryk Neethling, Olympic Swimmer and World Record Holder

I suggest every person who wants to maintain a healthy physical and mental state use E3Live on a daily basis. E3Live is a live food. You will easily digest and assimilate all the nutrients. E3Live is good for children, teenagers, and adults of any age.

—Dr. Theresa Dale, Ph.D., N.D.

I haven't had leg pains since the very first day of taking it and I had these pains for over 6 months without a break! It was keeping me from sleeping and making me grouchy. I've slept soundly and had ZERO leg pains.

—Raynee Steele

I am the CEO of a company and the stakes are high. If a telecom company goes off-line, it costs many thousands of dollars each minute! Since I began drinking E3Live, my engineers and colleagues have told me I'm more poised, focused and on-task. My threshold for handling stress has increased and my concentration is sharper. Solution-oriented resolutions to daily challenges come easier. Am I jazzed about E3Live? You better believe it!

—Bob Berry, President, DPS Telecom, One of *Inc. Magazine*'s Top 500 Fastest Growing Companies

Why Is Now the Best Time Ever to Try E3Live?

This is probably the first time you've heard of E3Live's incredible story, and you may still be a little skeptical. With that in mind, Vision has created what we believe is the most powerful guarantee in the natural-health industry. It says:

If you do not *Feel the Difference*—by your own evaluation—we will refund your purchase price (not including shipping) for up to one year.

So there's literally no risk to you! What's more, in conjunction with this publication, the folks at E3Live will "sweeten the pot" by giving you 20% OFF your first order of E3Live. (When you call our toll-free number, tell them *Natural Life News* sent you to get the discount.)

Still not convinced? Then call *Natural Life* [see *Natural Life*'s ad in Resources] to receive a CD with groundbreaking interviews by two of the country's top holistic doctors, along with an informative booklet and free samples of Vision's E3-AFA™ (dried AFA in vegetable capsules). Start TODAY by experiencing the life-changing health benefits that only E3Live offers! ▪

[EDITOR'S NOTE: **I offer this high-chlorophyll drink to all my clients prior to breathwork as an excellent way to boost their oxygen levels and prepare their body and blood for the healing work ahead.**]

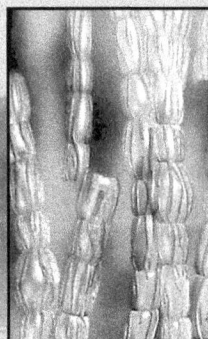

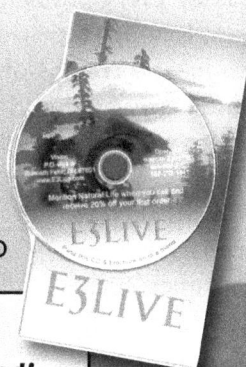

Nature's Solution to Cramping & Tetany

What can you do for those who suffer from nightly foot and leg cramps, for women with menstrual cramps or parents with a colicky baby, for athletes, dancers and other active people, for diabetics and those with restricted blood flow? Until now, there hasn't been much you could do. Now you can zap the cramp right out of their life with a tool straight from nature's pharmacy. The ZAP-A-KRAMP™ herbal pillow is fast, incredibly effective, safe and simple.

It has been said there's an herb for every problem of man. There is an herb that deals directly with muscle cramps of any type, located anywhere in the body (except those caused by a pinched or injured nerve). This herb has various names, such as common club moss and wolf's claw. The Latin name is *Lycopodium clavatum*. It is listed in the *American Pharmacopoeia of Homeopathic Remedies*. It works homeopathically by transferring the vibrational essence of the herb (contained in the pillow in its raw, ground, and undiluted form) directly into the muscle, enabling the muscle to relax. No side effects. Simply place the herbal pillow over the area of the cramp and relief begins in seconds. It works right through clothing. And it lasts for years!

The herb is so safe you can eat it, as the Chippewa Indians did, or you can steep it as a tea. It contains huperzine A, huperzine B, and the enzyme prolyl endopeptidase (PEP). These constituents of the tea help prevent the breakdown of acetylcholine, a neurotransmitter in the brain, which plays a key role in recognition, reasoning, and memory.

EDITOR's NOTE—This herb effectively relieves the tetany cramping that can occur during breathwork. However, my good friend Carlton Newman, founder of this company, has retired now and is no longer making these pillows. (I bought up his final batch and am using them to this day in my workshops.) Still, anyone can obtain wild-harvested club moss and use it for this purpose. IT REALLY WORKS!

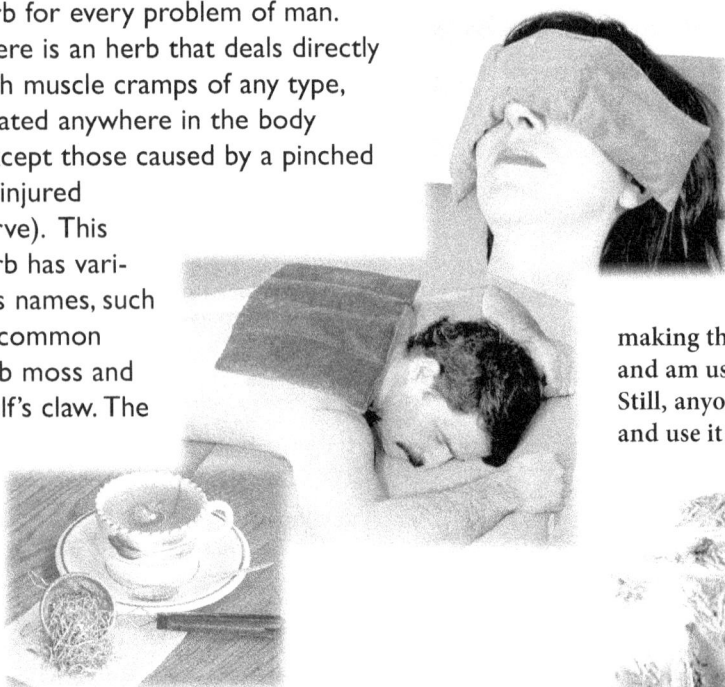

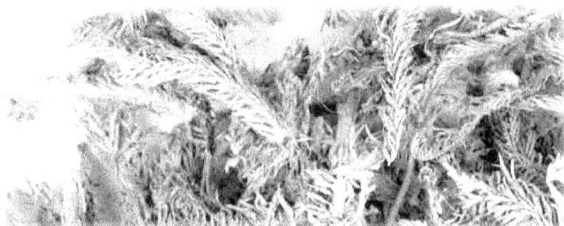

NATURAL LIFE NEWS

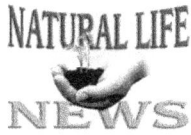

Natural & Holistic Self-Healing
METHODS ❖ EDUCATION ❖ DISCUSSION

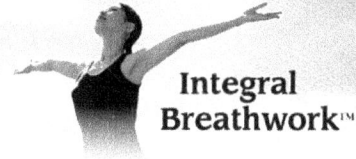

Integral Breathwork™

Home   From Editor   Magazine   Moringa   Herbs & Plants   Breathwork   E3Live   Book   Self-Publishing   Contact

Welcome to Natural Life News!

I believe everyone has the right and responsibility to take charge of their own healing. Doctors and medicine do their job, but when it comes to prevention, immune strength, vitality and freedom from pain, drugs and their side-effects, Nature does it better! You can heal yourself through the pure natural elements — air, water, sunlight, chlorophyll — the energy within these can awaken your body's natural healing abilities. Find out how... ~ Denis Ouellette

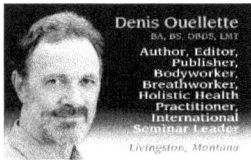

Denis Ouellette
BA, BS, DIBDS, LMT
Author, Editor, Publisher, Bodyworker, Breathworker, Holistic Health Practitioner, International Seminar Leader
Livingston, Montana

Insights
FROM THE EDITOR

With 35+ years in the healing arts practicing bodywork and holistic health, as a pioneer in breathwork development, and 15+ years of publishing Natural Life News, read here in Denis' own words his most fascinating stories and lessons learned.

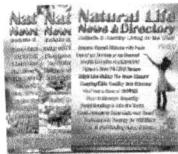

Natural Life News
ARCHIVES

Read and comment on the best articles from our magazine. Search by category. Our Archives go back 12+ years. We're always adding new posts. We feature experts in many fields of natural healing, delicious recipes, tips on psychology, financial health, etc.

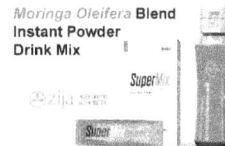

Moringa Oleifera **Blend Instant Powder Drink Mix**

"The Miracle Tree"
ZIJA'S MORINGA

Denis became a Zija Independent Distributor in the company's early days, when the great benefits of the Moringa Tree were first being discovered and developed. Read our foundational articles and become a part of Zija's worldwide health revolution!

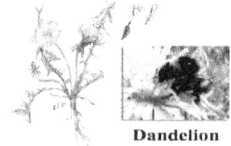

Dandelion

Native-American Uses of
HERBS & PLANTS

Elinora Stenersen Old Coyote
published 18 masterful articles on the ecology, Native-American folklore and uses of the herbs, trees and shrubs that are native to the Rockies and the great plains, spanning the Dakotas. Her invaluable life's work is here!

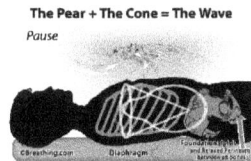

The Pear + The Cone = The Wave
Pause

INTEGRAL BREATHWORK
Stories • Seminars • Videos • Private Sessions

Breathwork is one of the greatest but least-known secrets of self-healing, producing astounding and almost miraculous results. An early pioneer (in the 1970s), with new understandings of its practice today, join Denis on his quest to bring breathwork to all.

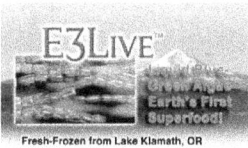

E3LIVE
Green Algae Earth's First Superfood!
Fresh-Frozen from Lake Klamath, OR

E3LIVE
Earth's First Food

In this day of nutritionally vacant foods, every body needs the vitality of Earth's first green superfood. This powerful, high-chlorophyll, blue-green algae blooms and is harvested from a pristine mountain lake in Oregon. Delivered fresh-frozen. The health benefits don't quit. Try it!

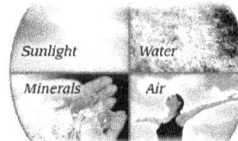

Sunlight   Water   Minerals   Air

HEAL YOURSELF
with Breath, Light, Sound & Water

Learn what full oxygenation, detoxification, and chi movement can do to cleanse and rejuvenate your body, mind, emotions and memories. Denis found the best natural-health teachers and interviewed them. His research spans decades but these practices span the timeless millennia.

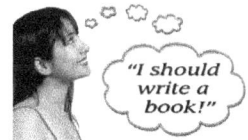

"I should write a book!"

SELF-PUBLISHING
Coaching & Services

Denis has assisted many first-time authors bring their raw manuscripts to beautiful, finished products, launching their careers. See samples of his work, visit with the published authors, and turn your dreams of getting published (in any genre) into a reality—on the fast track.

QUICK LINKS
› About
› Contact
› Subscribe to **Natural Life News**
› Get **Heal Yourself** Book
› Info/Ordering **Zija's Moringa**
› Order **E3Live** Samples

NEWSLETTER
Sign up to get occasional emails on our latest news.
Email Address*

First Name

* = required field

[Subscribe]

FREE BREATHING TEST
LEARN TO BREATHE BETTER NOW!

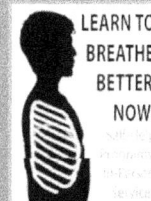

GRIEVING FOR A SISTER

The experience far exceeded my imagination. My sister and I thank you. I no longer have the painful pressure and trauma thoughts (flashbacks) that surrounded her death anymore. I only hear her laugh and see her smiles now. I still grieve the loss of her physical presence, but I feel better able to handle those moments as they come and go.

—Andy D. • Helena, MT

MY MOTHER'S FEAR FROM BIRTH

For the last several months, I've become more and more aware of how afraid I've become in everyday life. It seemed to be since I gave birth to my son (now almost 2). I would imagine some kind of catastrophe at the turn of every corner. As this awareness seemed to grow, I realized it was really inhibiting my happiness and creating unneeded stress.

During the breathwork session, I felt a numbness everywhere—the only place that seemed to finally release was around my jaw. I felt fear rising—a nameless, faceless fear. There were no images, and it seemed to be from the distant past. I kept breathing and I went through a second release. As people were starting to sit up, I calmed my breathing down and tried to come back to Earth. I felt I was zinging with energy—almost to the point of levitating off the floor! Finally, I was able to sit up, but I felt I had left something unfinished.

Two days later, I had an acupuncture appointment, which gave me the conclusion to my breathwork. As I was on the table, I started having a sensation I've had many times before... feeling like I'm breathing thick air, like water, and my very large head and small body seem to fill the entire space. I was returning to the womb. I thought of my mother telling me that she felt happy as long as I was in the womb where she could protect me, but she wasn't sure what would happen next, as she was giving me up for adoption. The feeling inside the womb was pure bliss—not a care in the world.

I realized then that my fear came from the moment of birth and not believing that the Universe was a loving place. I was feeding off my birth mother's own fear of what would happen to me when she was no longer there to protect me. In my mind, the newborn baby told my mother, "Look, I'm okay!" And I saw that I really was okay—the Universe IS a loving place! Since then, those doomsday scenarios have started to fade. If I do see one, out of habit, I see another scenario as well—of nothing out of the ordinary happening, and I tell myself that nothing dramatic happening could also be the probable course of events. And then I laugh. :-)

I called my birth mother, whom I've known for the last 23 years, and told her my story. She cried with joy—healing her young mother within as well!

—Margaux Murray • Montreal, March 28, 2009

A GRATEFUL FACILITATOR

The breathwork brought great healing and release on a very deep level to me. And Saturday evening, I realized that there had been additional shifting within me as a result of facilitating others. I find myself breathing throughout the day and even when awakening at night. It is becoming a part of me. What a true sharing of love! And how appreciative I am that my heart released such deep sorrow, and then filled with love as a result of this weekend. Thank you!

—Donna Rae • Libby, MT

RECONNECTED   HAPPY   SERENE

I GET TO BE ME!   ALIVE & FREE

WELL-BEING   RELAXED   LOOPY

PHENOMENAL   MORE PRESENT

MORE WHOLE   PERFECT

PEACEFUL   CONTENT   RADIANT

COMPLETE   DEEPER & FULLER

GRATEFUL   FREE   GROUNDED

FRESH   EXCITED   JOYFUL

I FEEL LIKE MYSELF AGAIN!

PROFOUND   QUIET   CLEARER

LIGHT & LOVE   ENERGIZED

WARM & TINGLY   COMFORTABLE

BLISS-CONNECTED   VIBRATING